Plandemic

Exposing the Greed, Corruption, and Fraud Behind the COVID-19 Pandemic

Dr. Bruce Fife

P B

Piccadilly Books, Ltd.
Colorado Springs, CO

Photo credits: page 28 Carl Fredrik Sjöland, Wikipedia Commons; page 31 Center for Disease Control and Prevention; page 42 ŽupaBA VUCBA, Wikipedia Commons.

Second Printing November 2020

Piccadilly Books, Ltd.
info@piccadillybooks.com
www.piccadillybooks.com

ISBN 9781936709298

Contents

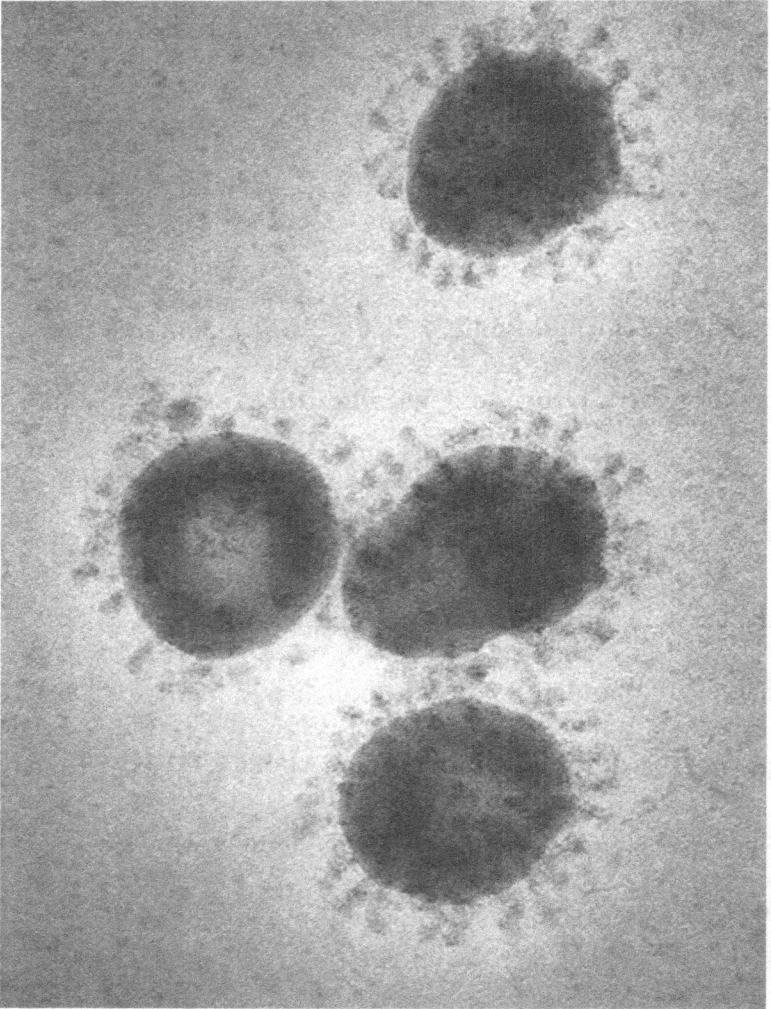

The coronavirus SARS-CoV-2.

1

The Outbreak

A NURSING HOME CALAMITY

The emergency dispatcher listened to the frantic caller: "Difficulty breathing...turning blue...come quickly!" Call after call came rolling in. Surprisingly, they all had the same address: 10101 NE 120th Street—Life Care Center nursing home in Kirkland, Washington—a suburb of Seattle. Within weeks two-thirds of Life Care's residents became ill; 35 of them died. The suspect? A newly discovered virus from China that was rapidly spreading worldwide.

News of the new virus was first released on December 31, 2019, when China reported a cluster of cases of pneumonia in people in the city of Wuhan. Seven days later Chinese health authorities confirmed that this outbreak was associated with a novel, or new, coronavirus similar to the one that caused the SARS outbreak in 2002-2003. Although initial cases were associated with exposure to a seafood market in Wuhan, epidemiologic data indicated that person-to-person transmission was occurring. Within one month a total of 9,976 cases were reported in at least 21 countries, including the first confirmed case in the United States. At the rate it was spreading it was expected to infect millions worldwide within months.

Life Care is not an unkempt, low rent nursing home, staffed by unskilled and underpaid workers, which might encourage the spread of disease. On the contrary, it is part of a nationwide chain of 200 facilities. The facility earned five stars out of five on its federal ratings for overall care the previous year. Families of the residents praised the workers and quality of care.

Many of the home's 120 residents were in their 80s or 90s, suffered from dementia, Parkinson's, emphysema, and other debilitating diseases and were living there permanently. Others were there for rehabilitation after an illness or surgery and, in time, hoped to return home. Most of the residents were taking multiple drugs to help them cope with their various health problems.

The 180 staff members included physicians, physical therapists, nurses, and nursing assistants, many of whom did the intimate work of bathing residents, getting them dressed, and lifting them out of bed to use the bathroom.

It was common for the residents to suffer from colds and flu and occasionally develop pneumonia, but the number of cases this season seemed higher than normal. Then came word that the coronavirus, the one in China that was all over the news, had hit in Kirkland. The first confirmed case in the US was reported just a few weeks earlier, also in the state of Washington.

On January 19, 2020, a 35-year-old man after experiencing a mild cough and low-grade fever for 4 days went to an urgent care clinic in Snohomish County, Washington. The clinic was less than 20 miles away from the Life Care Center nursing home in Kirkland. The man had returned to Washington on January 15 after traveling to visit family in Wuhan, China. Although his symptoms at the time were no worse than a typical cold, he was prompted to get a medical checkup after seeing a health alert from the US Centers for Disease Control and Prevention (CDC) about the novel coronavirus outbreak in Wuhan.

The medical examination revealed a history of hypertriglyceridemia, indicating an increased risk of heart disease, but otherwise he was in relatively good health. His blood pressure, heart rate, and other vital signs were all within normal range. A chest x-ray showed no signs of infection and he had no sinus discharge. He also tested negative for influenza A and B and for other known coronaviruses (SARS and MERS). Although the patient reported no known contact with ill persons during his travel to China, respiratory specimens were collected and sent to the CDC for analysis. On the following day, the CDC confirmed that the patient tested positive for COVID-19—the name given by the World Health Organization (WHO) for the new disease.

The patient was immediately isolated for observation and to prevent the spread of the disease. Under observation, the patient continued to cough and have a low-grade intermittent fever, which was followed by some abdominal discomfort and fatigue. He was given supportive therapy, such as Tylenol, to manage the symptoms, as well as supplemental oxygen. His symptoms were indistinguishable from many other common seasonal infectious diseases and his treatment was no different. After 8 days in the hospital (12 days of illness) the patient's clinical condition improved and symptoms were resolved. He was released a couple of days later.

The patient was apparently infected during his trip to China. He began to notice symptoms the day after he returned to Washington and sought medical attention 4 days later. During that time he could have passed the infection to others.

It is believed that employees or visitors, who may have thought they were simply fighting off a minor cold, brought the infection into the Life Care nursing home. Residents who are elderly, and generally in poor health, are extremely vulnerable to infections. Consequently, the virus ran rampant through the nursing home. At first, the staff was not surprised by a few patients with flu-like symptoms, as this was flu season and respiratory illness was common at this time of year. In early February, however, the staff began to get concerned as a larger than normal number of patients seemed to be coming down with what they believed was the flu. The flu season was in full swing and the number of flu cases during the

2019-2020 flu season had started out higher than usual. Other nursing homes in the area were also reporting higher than normal infection rates. Then, on February 26, two Life Care residents died, two days later, tests indicated the cause was COVID-19. More residents became ill.

The facility was immediately put on lockdown. The halls emptied. Bedroom doors were closed. Staff members, who felt ill or showed symptoms of illness, were told to stay home. Those that remained, had to pick up the slack, requiring them to work faster and stay longer as the workload increased.

One by one residents of the nursing home became sick. Initial symptoms included fever, tiredness, and dry cough. Some also experienced aches and pains, nasal congestion, runny nose, sore throat, and diarrhea. The symptoms were indistinguishable from other respiratory illnesses. According to the World Health Organization, some people don't develop any symptoms and don't feel sick. Fortunately, 95 percent of people over the age of 60 who get COVID-19 recover from the illness. A few, however, become seriously ill and develop breathing difficulties. The most vulnerable are older people and those with underlying health problems such as cardiovascular disease, diabetes, respiratory problems and high blood pressure. Those are the ones who are most likely to develop serious illness. Residents of nursing homes are at greatest risk and for this reason, the majority of cases were occurring in long-term care facilities.

Symptoms generally appear three to four days after exposure. Initially, the symptoms are mild and resemble a cold or flu, but can potentially progress to pneumonia. COVID-19 itself doesn't usually cause death, but a secondary bacterial or viral infection in the lungs can lead to pneumonia, which can be life threatening, especially among those with existing health problems, as is common in nursing homes.

In all, 129 people at Life Care, including 81 residents, tested positive for the virus, 35 of which died. Dozens of the center's employees were diagnosed with the coronavirus, suggesting that the frantic efforts to sanitize the building, quarantine residents, and shield staff members with gowns and masks, was ineffective. Essentially everyone in the nursing home—residents and staff alike—had been exposed to the virus.

Some of the health care employees at Life Care also worked at other nursing homes in the Seattle area. A few of the residents of Life Care were also transferred to other nursing homes at this time. CDC investigators determined that those who had been exposed to the virus at Life Care, carried it with them to other facilities, passing along the infection. Consequently, the infection spread to at least 23 other long-term care facilities in the area.

As with most seasonal respiratory illnesses, the coronavirus affects people differently. Some people show no signs or symptoms, others may develop mild or moderate symptoms, and still others may need to be hospitalized. At the Life Care nursing home the staff and residents were all exposed to the virus, most of whom showed only minor symptoms. They recovered. In contrast, elderly residents with underlying health problems, many of whom were taking multiple drugs, became very ill and were hospitalized or died. Why the difference? Why can two people exposed to the same virus have completely different responses?

Interestingly, at Life Care, more residents caught the virus and survived than those who died. Even though they were elderly and many suffered with serious chronic health issues, they were able to beat the disease. Out of the 81 residents who became sick, most of them, 46, recovered. In addition, 40 of the elderly residents did not become sick at all. Despite being just as old and vulnerable as the others, these residents showed no signs of illness, suggesting they were healthy enough to fight off the disease or that they already had immunity to the virus.

Respiratory infections in nursing homes are not restricted to pandemics but occur every year. We usually don't hear about them because they are a part of the ebb and flow of sea-

An Epidemic or a Pandemic?

Terms used to describe an outbreak can be confusing. What is the difference, if any, is there between an outbreak, epidemic, and pandemic? An outbreak is simply a sudden rise in cases of a disease in a particular place. An epidemic is a large outbreak that is confined to a specific geographical area. A pandemic means a global epidemic. Pandemic sounds scary but it has nothing to do with how serious the illness is. It just means a disease is spreading widely. A pandemic can be severe or mild. In 2009 the swine flu pandemic caused wide scale fear, like COVID-19, because it caused noticeable fatalities among high risk individuals, however, for most people it turned out to be a relatively mild illness.

sonal illness that occur worldwide. But it is long-term care facilities that are usually hit the hardest and provide the majority of the death statistics that are used to frighten everybody to encourage them to get their yearly flu vaccinations. For instance, during the 2017-2018 flu season the CDC estimates there were 61,000 deaths. The CDC reports the burden that year was "atypical in that it was severe for all ages." Of the hospitalizations for flu, 67 percent were in adults of nursing home age, who also accounted for 83 percent (50,630) of all deaths.[1]

The seasonal respiratory infections are most lethal to the elderly whose health is already challenged with chronic illness or who are immune compromised. Taking multiple drugs can also weaken the immune system. So when the coronavirus struck hospitals and nursing homes, the results were alarming. The number of people in nursing homes accounts for less than 1 percent of the US population, but accounted for a staggering 43.4 percent of all COVID-19 deaths[2] COVID-19 has little effect on children and young adults. Regardless of age, for the vast majority of the population those who have no serious underlying health problems, COVID-19 is no worse than a cold or the flu. Like most other seasonal viruses, an infection from the coronavirus produces long-term immunity to the virus in most people. This is the basis for the development of vaccines. When a person is exposed to certain viruses they produce antibodies that can make them immune to these viruses in the future. If we could not develop immunity, vaccines would be useless.

Our bodies are conditioned to fight off infection. We do it all the time, even when we are not aware of it. It is a constant battle with the microbes with which we share our environment. Whether it is a coronavirus, rhinovirus (cold), or influenza A or B, viruses are constantly around us. Nowhere are we totally free from exposure. Face masks won't prevent you from exposure, nor will social distancing. We are always exposed to potentially harmful viruses and bacteria. How vulnerable you are to infection depends on your health and the ability of your immune system to protect you.

AN INTERNTIONAL CRISIS
The events that occurred at Life Care nursing home were repeated in hundreds of long-term care facilities across the nation and throughout the world causing widespread alarm. The WHO proclaimed the outbreak to be a worldwide pandemic. Computer models predicted deaths would be in the millions. Daily the media reported the number of people infected and the accumulated death count. One by one nations around the world declared national health emergencies. Chinese officials locked down the city of Wuhan, shutting residents in their homes and forbidding travel in or out of the city in an effort to stop the spread of the virus. Other countries followed suit and enacted lockdowns and travel restrictions. By September 2020, we were told that COVID-19 had killed some 180,000 Americans.

The wearing of face masks, social distancing, closing of businesses and parks, banning of public gatherings and other drastic measures were mandated, often with the penalty of arrest or hefty fines for those who disobeyed. This was the first time in history that healthy individuals have been quarantined in order to prevent the spread of disease. It is also the first time countries have forcibly closed down businesses, banned people from going to work and making a living, except for government workers and a select few businesses deemed "essential," resulting in widespread economic and social turmoil for most citizens.

Was the pandemic as serious as the media and government health officials claimed? The facts don't fit the scenario we've been fed. The CDC admits the COVID-19 death count has been grossly overinflated. According to data released by the CDC, only 6 percent of all reported COVID-19 deaths could actually be attributed solely to the coronavirus.[3-4] Reported deaths from influenza and other respiratory infections virtually stopped after March 2020. The flu was rarely mentioned after that date. Did the flu suddenly cease to exist? Doctors reported COVID-19 fatalities on death certificates even when the patients' actual deaths were caused by influenza, heart attacks, cancer, and other fatal diseases as well as accidents, drug overdose, and suicide. Why were the COVID-19 deaths inflated? Why has the pandemic that crippled our economy and society been dramatically over-exaggerated? Why are the numbers used to justify all of the aggressive measures and taken away our freedoms so very wrong?

Never in the history of the world have government and health officials taken such drastic measures to combat an infectious disease. Why was this virus any different from previous outbreaks? Was it because it was more virulent, more contagious, or a greater threat? Or was there something else behind all the steps taken to address this particular outbreak at this particular time, something we are not being told? This book answers these questions and exposes the greed, corruption, and fraud behind the COVID-19 pandemic.

2

A Plandemic

The COVID-19 pandemic is not a naturally occurring outbreak like previous pandemics, but is a carefully orchestrated and planned event—a plandemic. The purpose is for a few organizations and businesses to gain global control, power, and wealth.

The true story of the COVID-19 pandemic plays out with the intrigue and corruption of a Hollywood suspense thriller. Except this story is shockingly true.

For some who have unquestionable faith in the honesty and integrity of government officials, drug companies, and public health authorities, it may be difficult to believe. To those who already recognize the corruption found in government and businesses regarding health and personal choice, it makes complete sense.

Everything stated in this book is true—all statements are referenced to their sources so that you can verify and confirm that they are not theories or fabrications of my own.

The information in this book is important because our health freedom is at stake of being taken away. We are being lied to in order to voluntarily give up our rights and freedom of choice in regards to making informed decisions about our health and the health of our families. We are encouraged and even compelled to surrender these choices to a few select individuals who hold positions of power and authority over us—individuals with morally questionable motives, with their own interests in mind, and little regard for us.

The purpose of this book is to expose the truth behind the COVID-19 plandemic so that you will be aware of the facts and not have your freedoms blindly taken from you. And empower you with knowledge so that you can make informed decisions regarding your own health and welfare.

FLATTENING THE CURVE

Contrary to the narrative projected by the mainstream media and public health officials, the COVID-19 pandemic did not start in Wuhan, China in December 2019, but began years earlier in boardrooms across the globe among some of the world's richest businessmen and women. Every step of the pandemic was carefully thought-out and planned to the tiniest detail, from the selection of the infectious agent (SARS-Cov-2) to its method of release, and how it would be publically promoted to generate the greatest amount of fear and panic. The exact steps taken to manage the plandemic were designed to maximize the world's fear and make us more vulnerable, all in the guise of prevention or as they call it to "flatten the curve."

Never before in history has governments worldwide closed down their countries, stopped citizens from going to work and making a living, or isolate themselves in their homes. And for what? Simply to flatten the curve. We've heard this term over and over again but what does it mean to "flatten the curve"? Most of us tend to believe it is a means to reduce the spread of the virus so that fewer people become infected, but that is absolutely wrong! It does not mean to reduce the number of people infected—it simply means to extend or slow down the spread of the disease so that not as many people become sick at the same time. If you would have become sick without these measures, you

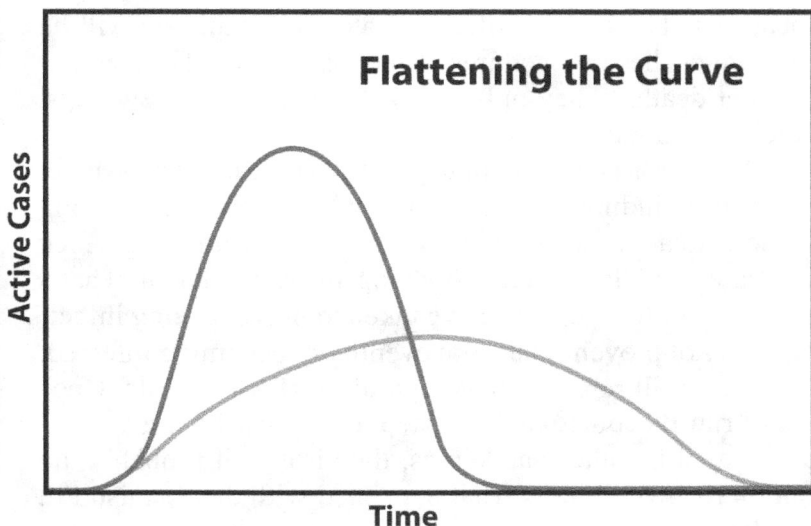

Flattening the Curve

Active Cases (y-axis)

Time (x-axis)

The purpose for flattening the curve is not to prevent people from getting sick, but to slow down the rate of infection to avoid a peak that would overwhelm hospitals and healthcare workers. The measures to fatten the cure are not meant to prevent infection, only delay it. The same total number of people will still eventually be infected.

will still eventually become sick. Your ultimate risk of dying is the same regardless of whether you follow the mandates or not. It only prolongs the duration of the outbreak. The justification for flattening the cure is not to prevent you from getting sick or to save lives, it is to prevent hospitals and healthcare workers from being overwhelmed by a possible sudden onslaught of cases over a short period of time.

Social distancing, wearing of masks, closing of businesses, parks, sporting events and churches, and the insistence on excessive sanitation procedures, etc. that we have been instructed and mandated to follow are done to flatten the curve—not to prevent anyone from getting sick or from dying. The idea that flattening the curve saves lives is a myth perpetuated by government officials and health administrators to compel you to comply to all of their insane measures. The overall infection rate and death rate will be the same. These procedures do not save lives. They do not prevent deaths. They only delay the deaths by a few days, weeks, or months.

This virus is highly contagious and spreads everywhere. There is no hiding from it. It will find you. If you are among those who are susceptible to it, you will eventually get sick regardless of the social distancing measures taken. That's right! All of the steps we have taken to prevent being infected, will not prevent you from eventually becoming infected. The virus will run its course regardless of what we do. Once it has run its course and infected all those who are vulnerable, just like other pandemics, the virus will probably die out on its own. That is what happened with the Spanish Flu pandemic of 1918, the most deadly viral outbreak in recorded history. Once it ran its course, it disappeared. The same is true with other viruses. We cannot stop this new virus. It will run its course regardless of what we do.

Think of that. the measures we have been taking, contrary to popular belief, will not save a single life! Everything we hear about saving lives to compel us to follow the social distancing rules is a lie. The shaming and persecution thrown on those who can think for themselves and choose not to follow these senseless regulations will not change things. Social distancing does not save lives or prevent the spread of the virus.

The only possible benefit is that it may delay the infection in some people long enough for a vaccine to be developed and for everyone to be vaccinated. That is the real goal. However, by the time an effective vaccine is developed, most everyone who would be infected will be before a vaccine is available.

A NOVEL VIRUS

In order for the plandemic to work, it had to be caused by a "novel" or new virus, one in which no one had immunity. Therefore, everyone on earth would be potentially vulnerable and would infect millions worldwide. But new human viruses that are highly contagious and have the potential to kill, just don't come along all that often. One option would be a virus that had already caused worldwide panic in previous years but had died out naturally, such as the Spanish flu of 1918 or the Asian flu of 1957, one that occurred so long ago most people would not have an immunity to it. Such a virus would need to be "accidentally" released from a research lab. However, this might cause some animosity against viral research using known highly pathogenic viruses that have been kept around.

A better plan is to find a virus that is completely new, one that would not have any existing antivirals or vaccines to fight it, requiring the development of new, and expensive, drugs to treat it. It would be a ticket to great wealth for drug makers and shareholders. Such a virus may be the product of genetic mutations that allow a deadly animal virus to jump to a human host. This type of research is being done all over the world. It would be relatively easy to find a suitable virus and have it secretly released so that it appears to be the result of a natural processes of transferring from animals to humans—a process that is known to happen. No one would be the wiser.

The SARS (SARS-CoV) coronavirus was a perfect candidate. It was responsible for the SARS outbreak in 2002, which was highly fatal. A number of labs throughout the world had been studying this virus, some of which were investigating how it could become more contagious and more lethal. Such a virus would be ideal for a pandemic. The result was the novel SARS-CoV-2 virus, the cause of COVID-19.

3

The Origin of COVID-19

THE EMERGENCE OF A NEW DISEASE

In early December 2019, doctors and nurses in Wuhan, China were puzzled to see a cluster of patients with symptoms of a viral pneumonia that did not respond to the usual treatments. By December 20 the number of patients with the mysterious illness climbed to 60. The symptoms of this illness resembled SARS—a potentially fatal respiratory illness caused by a coronavirus. Doctors were concerned because SARS originated in China and caused a massive outbreak in 2002. The virus spread to numerous countries, killing hundreds of people. Doctors were worried that they may be witnessing a new SARS outbreak.

On December 24, doctors sent samples for analysis. Two days later, the results came back; it was not SARS but a new SARS-like coronavirus. The report was also sent to the Chinese health authorities in Beijing. The Chinese government, however, kept silent, hoping to contain the disease before it became public knowledge. The mishandling of the earlier 2002 SARS epidemic was an embarrassment to them and they did not want a repeat performance. Chinese authorities put secrecy and censorship ahead of openly confronting the growing crisis and risking public alarm or political embarrassment. By December 30, at least 266 people had been infected, but still there was no warning of the pending pandemic.

Concerned that this could be the beginning of another SARS outbreak, Dr. Li Wenliang alerted some of his medical colleagues in a private WeChat group. He told them of 7 patients who worked at the Huanan market in Wuhan who were quarantined in the emergency department at the hospital with the initial diagnosis of SARS. Although he requested confidentiality from those he shared the information, rumors of a deadly SARS outbreak spread quickly on Chinese social media.

It is believed that the SARS epidemic of 2002 occurred when a coronavirus jumped from bats to masked palm civets, a catlike creature that is legally raised and consumed and was sold in Chinese markets. It was likely that the new coronavirus had followed a similar path, possibly from food or animals sold at the Huanan market.

On January 1, 2020 police officers showed up at the market, along with public health officials, and shut it down. Local officials issued a notice that the market was undergoing an environmental and hygienic cleanup related to the pneumonia outbreak. That morning, workers in hazmat suits moved in, washing out stalls and spraying disinfectants. This was the first visible government response to contain the disease. Yet, no warning was issued to the citizens of Wuhan or reports sent to the World Health Organization (WHO) and other health agencies.

Nine days after the market closed, an elderly man who shopped at the Huanan market regularly became the first fatality of the disease. Unlike those who had recovered earlier, he already suffered from chronic liver disease and a tumor in his abdomen when he checked into the Wuahn Puren Hospital with a raging fever and difficulty breathing.

After Dr. Li's warning to his colleagues, which was shared on the internet, began to attract more attention the supervision department of his hospital summoned him for a talk. He was reprimanded and blamed for leaking the infor-

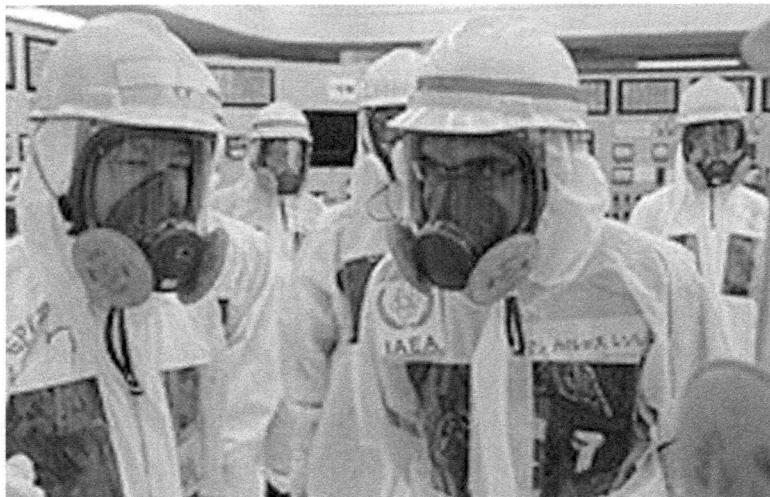

Workers in hazmat suits cleaned and sanitized the Huanan market, yet the government still did not warn people of the growing outbreak.

mation. On January 3, 2020, police from the Wuhan Public Security Bureau investigating the case interrogated Li and forced him to sign a confession stating that his remarks were untrue and constituted "illegal behavior." He was compelled to say nothing more about it or face prosecution. Li returned to work at the hospital and later contracted the disease from an infected patient and died. Since the government wasn't doing it, other doctors sounded the alarm as well and they too were reprimanded and silenced for spreading "rumors."

Word of the outbreak spread. Chinese officials insisted the disease was not spreading through human contact and that in a few days the outbreak would be over. The World Health Organization's statements during this period echoed the reassuring words of Chinese officials. The Director General of WHO, Tedros Adhanom Ghebreyesus, praised the way China was handling the situation, reassuring us that they were doing everything possible to contain the outbreak. We had nothing to worry about.

The Chinese government's initial denial of the epidemic and the WHO's inaction allowed the virus to spread to other parts of China and into neighboring countries. On January 13, 2020 the first case outside China was reported in Thailand. By January 30, 2020 there were a total of 7,818 confirmed cases reported worldwide, with the majority of these in China, and 82 cases reported in 18 countries outside China, including North America and Europe. The first confirmed death was in Wuhan on January 9, 2020. The first death outside China was on February 1 in the Philippines and the first death outside Asia was in France on February 14. The speed at which the virus spread indicated that it was highly contagious and on March 11 the WHO officially declared it to be a worldwide pandemic. Within days, national emergencies were declared in North America, Europe, and elsewhere.

THE NEW CORONAVIRUS

This new virus belongs to a family of coronaviruses that have caused two major multi-country epidemics that had occurred over the past 18 years. The new virus is closely related to an older coronavirus known as SARS-CoV, or simply SARS, which has a frightening fatality rate of 9.5 percent. In contrast, the annual flu has an average death rate of only 0.1 percent. If this new viruses was anything like its older cousin, it was something to be definitely worried about.

The new virus was named SARS-CoV-2. The World Health Organization named the illness caused by the new virus COVID-19, an acronym for "coronavirus disease 2019." The 2019 designates the year in which the virus was first identified.

The virus is believed to be spread primarily between people in close contact with each other, most often by small droplets produced by coughing, sneezing, and talking. The droplets usually fall to the ground or onto surfaces rather than travelling through air over long distances.[1] Less commonly, people may become infected by touching contaminated surfaces and then touch their face. A person is most contagious during the first three days after the onset of symptoms. Initially it was believed, or at least promoted, that the virus could be passed to others before symptoms were evident, but this theory has since been shown to be false. Unfortunately, many of the measures taken to flatten the cure and slow the spread of the virus are based on the erroneous theory that asymptomatic people—those who are infected but display no symptoms—are the primary carriers of the disease.

When the COVID-19 outbreak first occurred, it was often referred to as the "novel" coronavirus. Any virus that is new or very different from current and recently circulating human viruses are referred to as "novel." Such viruses when they infect humans have the potential to cause a pandemic because nobody has experienced them before so nobody has developed immunity to them. Everyone is vulnerable and so a new virus spreads easily and rapidly. Once people have been exposed to the virus, if it returns, it spreads much slower and infects fewer people. Since the characteristics of new viruses are unknown, how virulent they may be is also unknown. There is always the danger that they could cause serious disease and death. For this reason, new viruses are always viewed with caution and trepidation. Predictions and warnings are often overstated, but it is best to error on the side of caution than be caught by surprise and be unprepared. To get an idea of the severity of the disease, using what data was available at the time, the fatality rate was estimated to be as high as 4 percent or 40 times more deadly than the flu. Because there were no proven medications or vaccines available at the time, people were in a panic.

Unfortunately, when outbreaks occur, the media is quick to exploit the situation through sensationalism and fearmongering. News outlets with the most dramatic news stories tend to get the largest exposure and earn the most from advertising and sales. Such reporting creates widespread concern and fear, which in turn, encourages the media to pump out more shocking stories and dire warnings that outdo the previous reports, which can lead to greater fear and panic. The resulting hysteria can lead to irrational thinking and behavior, such as buying and hording massive amounts of toilet paper, hand sanitizer, and medicines, leaving store shelves bare for weeks or months.

According to Maciej Boni of Penn State University, "Left unchecked, infectious outbreaks typically plateau and then start to decline when the disease runs out of available hosts. But it's almost impossible to make any sensible projection right now about when that will be."[2] The WHO said the pandemic could be controlled by adhering to some dramatic changes in our normal day-to-day activities. Physical distancing, wearing of face masks, self-isolation, and other measures will be required until a vaccine becomes available, we were told.[3] William Schaffner of Vanderbilt University said because the coronavirus is "so readily transmissible," it "might turn into a seasonal disease, making a comeback every year."[4] A COVID-19 vaccine would become another one of the many annual vaccines promoted each year. The degree to which it might return each year would depend on herd immunity, so everyone would be encouraged, and possibly even mandated by law, to be vaccinated.

Countries worldwide went into lockdown in an effort to slow down the spread of the virus. By March 26, 1.7 billion people worldwide were under some form of lockdown, which increased to 3.9 billion people by the first week of April—more than half the world's population.[5] Tight travel restrictions were put into place, unless a person's job was essential for the welfare of the community, people were told to stay home. People could leave home only to perform essential services or shop for food, medicine, and other necessities. This was the first time in history that countries throughout the world shut down to stem the spread of a disease. The resulting shutdown, caused many business to close (some temporarily and some permanently), and workers to be laid off, causing the worst worldwide economic recession since the Great Depression.

4

The Coronavirus

CORONAVIRUSES AND THE COMMON COLD

Coronaviruses are a family of RNA (ribonucleic acid) viruses. Some strains can be transmitted between animals and humans, but most strains cannot. In humans, they cause respiratory illness with symptoms that can range from those resembling a mild cold to life threatening.

There are four human coronaviruses (HCoV) that have been around for a long time: HCoV-NL63, HCoV-229E, HCoV-OC43, and HCoV-HKU1. These viruses cause only a mild upper respiratory infection and are considered to be among those viruses that cause the common cold. They account for about 10 to 30 percent of the incidents attributed to the common cold. Like rhinoviruses (another cause of the common cold) and influenza, they appear seasonally each year and are found worldwide.

All of these respiratory viruses tend to cycle seasonally, appearing in winter and nearly disappearing in the summer. Coronaviruses are killed by modest heat and sunlight and thrive in dark environments. People tend to go outdoors more during the spring and summer, become more active, breathe fresh air, eat more fresh fruits and vegetables, and get exposure to sunshine that triggers the formation of vitamin D, all of which strengthens immune function and promotes better overall health. In winter, people are generally less active and in close confinement in buildings where infections can easily spread. This is why flu season occurs during the winter months and then fades as summer approaches. The best thing you can do during flu season is to spend time outside, which has been discouraged during the COVID-19 pandemic and has undoubtedly increased people's susceptibly to the infection. It almost seems like these lockdowns and harsh restrictions were put into place to make us more vulnerable to the virus. But why would anyone want people to get sick? The only ones who would benefit would be those selling cold and flu medications and other drugs, tissues, sanitizers, face masks, testing kits, and when available, antivirals and vaccines.

NEW BREED OF CORONAVIRUS

Since 2002, three new coronavirus (CoV) have surfaced (SARS-CoV, SARS-CoV-2, and MERS-CoV), which have proven to be far more troublesome. When they first appeared, each provoked large-scale epidemics, spreading quickly to numerous countries, causing multiple deaths. However, only the latest, SARS-CoV-2, was officially declared a pandemic by the World Health Organization. SARS—an acronym for "severe acute respiratory syndrome"—is a potentially fatal condition that is accompanied by severe coughing, labored breathing, and pneumonia or even severe acute respiratory syndrome, depending on the health status and age of the patient.

The first of the three to appear, SARS-CoV, known simply as SARS, surfaced in Guangdong, China in 2002. The epidemic quickly spread to at least 2 dozen countries, lasted 8 months, resulting in approximately 8,098 confirmed cases with 774 deaths (9.5 percent mortality rate). The virus seems to have run its course as no new cases have been reported for several years. MERS-CoV, known as MERS (Middle East respiratory syndrome) surfaced in 2012 in Saudi Arabia, spread to 27 countries, infecting 2,260 people resulting in 803 deaths (35.5 percent mortality).[1] Outbreaks were confined primarily to hospitals infecting immune-compromised patients. Since the 2012 outbreak, smaller outbreaks have occurred in following years in the Middle East and Asia. Although MERS continues to be a low level public health threat, there is concern that the virus could mutate to exhibit increased person-to-person transmission, with pandemic potential.

Although the third coronavirus, COVID-19, spread to nearly every country in the world and infected several million people, killing thousands, the death rate has been estimated to be between 0.05 and 0.1 percent of those infected. While COVID-19 is not nearly as deadly as SARS or MERS, it is far more contagious and thus able to infect many more people, putting more people at risk.

Prior to 2002, coronaviruses were thought to only cause disease in certain animals and mild colds in humans. However, when SARS emerged in China in 2002 it demonstrated that these viruses have the potential to cause serious widespread epidemics.

Coronaviruses are believed to have originated in horseshoe bats, from which over 200 species of coronavirus have been identified. The virus has an amazing ability for cross-species transmission. The mechanism for virus transmission from infected bats to livestock and humans is still unknown. There is evidence that there are seasonal fluctuations in virus replication, with peak activity in the spring, during which time threat of infection is greatest.[2] The coronaviruses in bats cannot be directly transferred to us, therefore, they require an intermediate host before spreading to humans. It is believed that SARS was passed to humans through contact with infected masked palm civets.

The SARS virus has been found in masked palm civets sold in live-animal markets in Guangdong, China. Another possible carrier is the raccoon dog, a small fox-like animal, also sold at these markets. Since cooking kills the virus, it is believed to have infected humans after they had eaten or handled raw or undercooked meat from these animals or by contact with their saliva, mucus, urine, or feces.

MERS, which is also known as the camel flu, is believed to have been spread from bats to humans by infected camels in the Middle East, where people are often in close contact with camels and also eat and drink their meat and milk.[3] In studying the origin of MERS, researchers were surprised to find that many camels carried viruses related to HCoV-229E, one of the coronaviruses that cause the common cold, suggesting that sometime in the past this virus also was passed to humans by contact with camels.[4] HCoV-229E has spread worldwide and is among the seasonal cold viruses that appear every year. The discovery of this virus in camels has caused concern that with slight genetic modification, MERS could do the same.

Like SARS and MERS, it is generally believed that SARS-CoV-2 originated in horseshoe bats; however, it is unlikely that the virus jumped directly from bats to humans based on what's known about transmission of coronaviruses. Instead, scientists suspect that the bat coronavirus jumped to another animal, an intermediate host, which subsequently transmitted the virus to humans.

Patients who first came down with COVID-19 in Wuhan all had contact with the Huanan Seafood Wholesale Market—a local "wet" market in the city. These markets consist of numerous small stalls crammed closely together selling live fish, poultry, red meat, and wild game. The term "wet" becomes obvious if you visit one. Live fish and crustaceans in open tubs splash water on the floor. The countertops in the stalls are red with blood as fish are gutted and filleted in front of the customers. The tables are rinsed

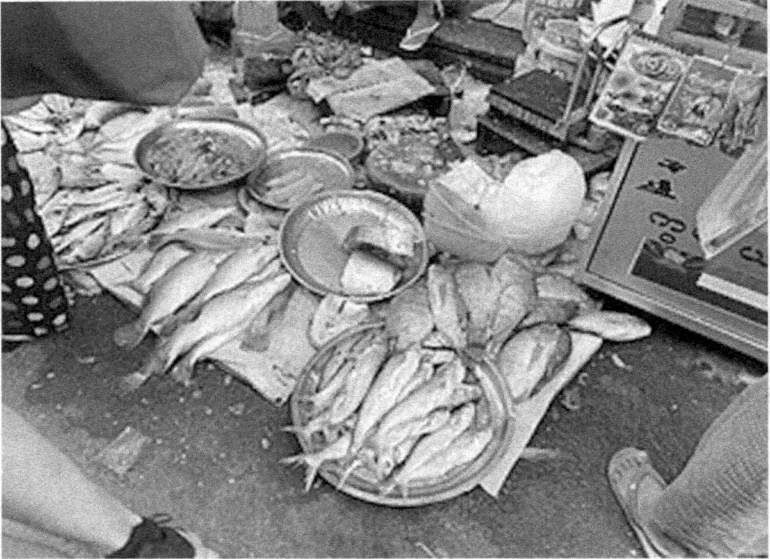
Wet market with fish on display for sale.

with water between customers. Live turtles, lobsters, and chickens climb over each other in tanks and cages. Lots of water, melting ice, and animal guts and waste cover the floor. Things are wet.

In China, exotic animals, some of which may not be native to that part of Asia, such as pangolins and peacocks, are considered delicacies and are often believed to provide special health-promoting properties. Many of these animals are sold live and butchered at the market. In such environments domestic and exotic animals are kept in close contact with each other and may transfer viruses from one species to another. In addition, viruses commonly share DNA leading to the development of new strains. It is generally believed that SARS-CoV-2 was transmitted to humans from animals sold at these markets.

LAB GENERATED CORONAVIRUS
Cover-up

There is a second theory on the origin of SARS-CoV-2 that gets little attention by the mainstream media, likely due to censorship by the powers behind the pandemic. The second possibility, as disturbing as it may be, is that SARS-CoV-2 is not a natural virus at all but was developed in a lab and accidentally leaked in Wuhan due to unsafe laboratory practices. An even more creepy possibility is that the virus was purposely released. In either case, a substantial amount of evidence points to the virus coming from a lab.

Infectious organisms studied in laboratories around the world are rated by their containment level (CL). The higher the level, the more barriers there are to prevent the escape of pathogens. If one fails, the next should ensure there is no danger. CL1 and CL2 labs work on fairly benign organisms. More dangerous pathogens, such as those that cause anthrax, plague, and rabies, can be handled in secure CL3 labs. The most dangerous and often exotic organisms, such as Ebola, Marbug, and Lassa viruses must be handled in CL4 labs. These organisms can kill, spread easily, and are often untreatable.

Wuhan is the home of China's highest-security virology research facility—the Wuhan Institute of Virology (WIV). WIV houses the Wuhan National Biosafety Laboratory, which is China's only Biosafety CL4 lab. That means it is the only facility in China permitted to handle the most dangerous pathogens.

It is possible that the novel coronavirus was being studied at WIV and an accident or a breech in lab safety protocol resulted in the virus' accidental transmission to an employee who then unknowingly spread the virus in the city after leaving the institute premises. Breaches in lab safety in China and elsewhere have occurred in the past at other research facilities. In the UK, for example, where safety precautions are well maintained, over 100 incidents occurred over a 5-year period that could have spread into the community some of the world's most deadly pathogens, including anthrax and Ebola. In one case, scientists mistakenly shipped live anthrax to other labs in the UK and North America. They meant to send harmless samples, killed by heat. But somehow the tubes got mixed up. Instead of sending dead bacteria, the anthrax was live and deadly. The recipients were unaware of the danger and opened the tubes without taking needed precautions.[5] This isn't just a problem in the UK but occurs worldwide wherever there are level 3 and 4 biosafety labs.[6]

In some cases, security breaches are done purposely, as was a case in July 2019 that occurred at the Canadian National Microbiology Laboratory (NML) in Winnipeg,— Canada's equivalent to the US Center for Disease Control and Prevention (CDC). A group of Chinese virologists working at the NML were forcibly evicted on suspicion of espionage for China. The scientists had been involved in the Special Pathogen Program of Canada's public health agency. One of the procedures conducted by the team was the infection of monkeys with the most lethal viruses found on earth. Four months prior to the Chinese team's eviction, an unauthorized shipment containing two exceptionally virulent viruses—Ebola and Nipah—was sent from the NML to a lab in China. Several of the researchers had been involved in Chinese biological weapons development. The senior scientist of the group, Xiangguo Qiu, who focused on Ebola research, had been in collaboration with Chinese bioweapons laboratories. The shipment of the two viruses from NML to China is alarming in itself, but it also raises the question of what other shipments of viruses or bacteria might have been made to China during the years she worked at the NML?[7]

Although the Wuhan Institute of Virology was a level 4 facility, security there, as it often is in other Chinese

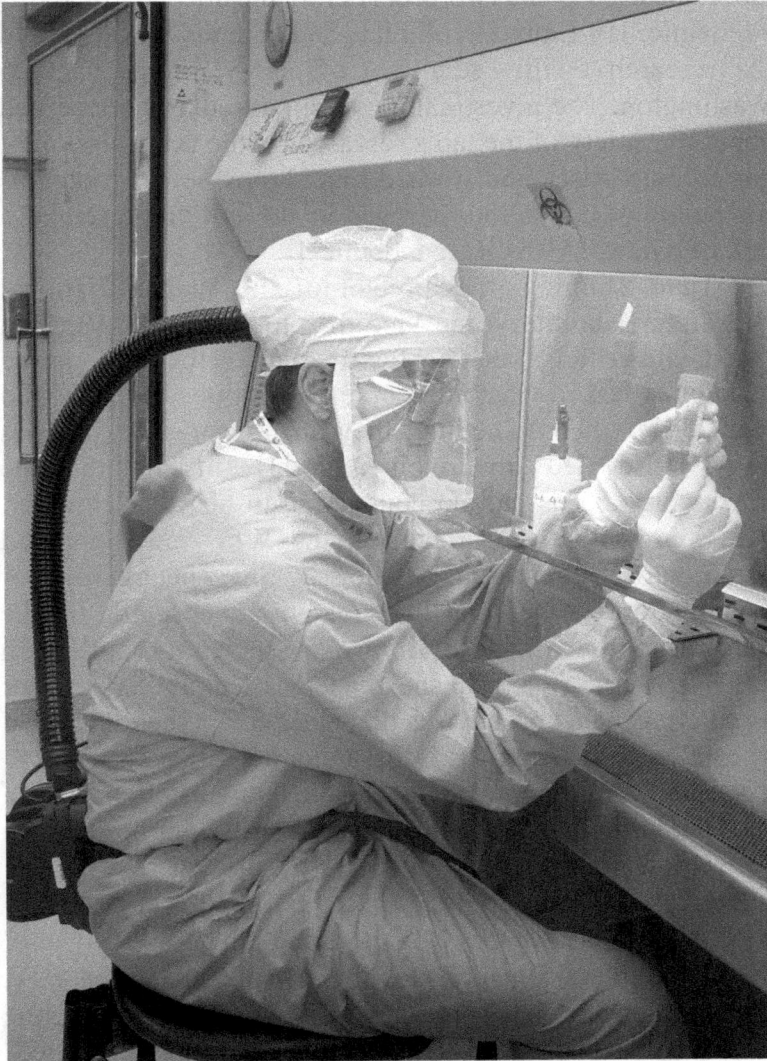

A microbiologist at the CDC biosafety level-3 enhanced lab examining reconstructed 1918 pandemic influenza virus contained in a vial. Scientists working with harmful pathogens wear a flow hood, which filters out any microorganisms that may escape into the atmosphere inside the laboratory.

laboratories, is poor. Two years before the novel coronavirus pandemic, US Embassy officials and scientists who visited the research facility sent two official warnings back to Washington. The investigators were particularly concerned about the safety of the lab's research on the transmission of bat coronaviruses and warned that sloppy safety protocols for handling contagious viruses in the lab "represented a risk of a new SARS-like pandemic."[8]

Yuan Zhiming, the director of the Wuhan National Biosafety Laboratory and vice director of the WIV, when faced with criticism that his facility may be the origin of the pandemic, he did what all people in positions of leadership tend to do when something they are responsible for goes awry. He denied any involvement. He insisted that the novel coronavirus had no connection to his lab. However, it is known that researchers at the WIV were involved in coronavirus research. Virologist, Shi Zhengli, one of the directors at the WIV had been doing research on the transmissibility of SARS from one species to another. In 2013 it is reported that she made a breakthrough in her research using a coronavirus that was 96.2 percent identical to SARS-CoV-2.[9] In 2015 she announced that the SARS-like virus could jump from bats to humans. It has been speculated that the new coronavirus came from her lab. An accusation she denies.

At a news conference on May 3, 2020, US Secretary of State, Mike Pompeo announced that SARS-Cov-2 originated in a bioweapons lab in Wuhan, China—the WIV. Speaking on the ABC program "This Week," Pompeo, the former CIA chief, said that "there's enormous evidence" that the coronavirus came from the lab, but at the time did not go so far as to claim that the virus was man-made or genetically modified.

When pressed for evidence he said that he was not allowed to give that information. It was later revealed that at least some of the evidence came from electronic intercepts of communications among Chinese officials. Realizing they were at fault for releasing this virus onto the world, government officials at all levels tried to hide the truth by censoring the media and punishing doctors for spreading "rumors."

Pompeo repeatedly accused China's Communist Party, led by President Xi Jinping, of covering up evidence and denying American experts access to the research lab at Wuhan. "We've seen the fact that they kicked the journalists out," Pompeo said, referring to orders that American correspondents from The New York Times, The Washington Post, and The Wall Street Journal leave China. "We saw the fact that those who were trying to report on this, medical professionals inside of China, were silenced. They shut down reporting—all the kind of things that authoritarian regimes do, the way Communist parties operate."[10] Why all the secrecy and denial? Perhaps they have something to hide—like the fact that they have been secretly working on bioweapons development, which has been banned by international law. Now it makes more sense why Chinese authorities were so adamant about censoring information about the outbreak and why they didn't admit the potential danger or take action until after it became international news.

The Chinese government has vigorously denied that the virus leaked from the laboratory. Both Chinese and international news reporters have been bared or censored from reporting on the incident in Wuhan. In an attempt to distract attention from China's own censorship and mismanagement in the early weeks of the epidemic and direct it toward someone else, Chinese officials claimed that the American military created it.[11]

Chinese government officials went to considerable lengths to cover up evidence about the outbreak and detained scientists who warned about it. A total lockdown on information related to the virus origins was put in place.

Beijing refused to provide US experts with samples of the novel coronavirus collected from the earliest cases. They closed a laboratory in Shanghai after one of its lead scientists shared the genomic sequence of the virus with collaborators around the world. That data has been critical to medical research, including on possible vaccines, but the Chinese authorities said the laboratory had to be closed down for "rectification."[12] Several of the doctors and journalists who reported on the spread early on have disappeared.

Gain-of–Function Research

Biosafety labs in the US have been doing research on coronaviruses for several years, including "gain-of-function" research intended to make pathogens more deadly and more transmissible. Such research involves manipulating viruses in the lab to explore their potential for infecting humans and provide clues to make better vaccines. Many scientists have criticized gain-of-function research because it creates a risk of starting a pandemic from accidental release. In October 2014, all federal funding was halted on any pathogen that could potentially cause a pandemic. The ban, however, was lifted in December 2017.

Dr. Anthony Fauci, who heads the National Institute for Allergy and Infectious Disease (NIAID), has served as an adviser to every US president since 1984. He has been the chief advisor to the White House in its response to the COVID-19 pandemic. Oddly enough, Dr. Fauci's comments and recommendations during the pandemic have often been contradictory and, in some cases, absurd, such as his insistence that lockdowns continue, sporting events be canceled, and schools and universities be closed until a vaccine is available. We must have a vaccine first he insists before things can get back to normal. Although he promotes social distancing and wearing of masks, he has stated that having sex with a stranger is ok.[13] It makes you wonder if his vaccine patents and close relationship with the pharmaceutical industry has any influence with his opinions.[14]

Having Fauci as the medical advisor during this pandemic is like having a fox guarding the hen house. Fauci is a long time supporter of gain-of-function research. He is aware of the risks, but feels it is justified in the search for new vaccines.

A decade ago, during a controversy over gain-of-function research on bird flu viruses, Dr. Fauci played an important role in promoting the work. He argued that the research was worth the risk because it enables scientists to make preparations, such as investigating possible anti-viral medications, that could be useful if and when a pandemic occurred.

The work in question was a type of gain-of-function research that involved taking wild viruses and passing them through live animals until they mutate into a form that could pose a pandemic threat. Scientists used it to take a virus that was poorly transmitted among humans and make it into one that was highly transmissible—a hallmark of a pandemic virus. This work was done by infecting a series of ferrets, allowing the virus to mutate until a ferret that hadn't been deliberately infected contracted the disease.

The work entailed risks that worried even seasoned researchers. More than 200 scientists called for the work to be halted. The problem, they said, is that it increased the likelihood that a pandemic would occur through a laboratory accident.

In 2014 with the backing of Fauci and the NIAID, the National Institutes of Health committed $3.7 million for research that included gain-of-function projects. Although the ban on funding gain-of-function research began in 2014, it did not stop this type of work. The National Institutes of Health allowed the controversial research to continue if the research had begun before the ban was put in place. Therefore, a portion of that grant money was used to fund

Shi Zhengli's coronavirus research at the Wuhan lab. An additional $3.7 million was granted at the beginning of 2020, which included gain-of-function research for the purpose of understanding how bat coronaviruses could mutate to attack humans.[15]

It appears very plausible, and even likely, that SARS-Cov-2 came from the Wuhan Institute of Virology. There is also another possibility. The management of the COVID-19 pandemic and the overemphasis on the importance and even necessity of having a vaccine to fight it, strongly suggests the pharmaceutical industry's hand in the way the crisis has been perceived and managed. Many suspect the drug industry had a major role to play in this crisis. The timing and steps taken have been too precise to attribute it to chance. If the drug companies are somehow involved, it is possible that they initiated the entire event. In this scenario, an employee at the Wuhan Institute of Virology who had access to the new virus in Shi Zhengli's lab could have been bribed to purposely release it somewhere in Wuhan, perhaps at the wet market. The Huanan market is only 9 miles from the institute. Released among raw fish, meats, and other foods, in a heavily trafficked market would be the ideal place to start a pandemic. Most of the initial cases were people who worked or shopped at the market.

5

Fear and Panic

PROMOTING FEAR AND PANIC

In early 2020 the world was thrown into a panic, fearful of being infected or infecting others with a previously unknown pathogen that has been portrayed as a highly contagious and lethal virus that has left thousands of victims dead worldwide. Along with confusion and uncertainty, we were also traumatized by the authoritarian measures governments have taken in response to the COVID-19 pandemic. Public health and government officials, as well as many citizens, were all clamoring for a vaccine to save us all from this terrible menace so that life could return to normal.

What most people do not realize is that much of the fear and panic associated with the COVID-19 pandemic was cleverly planned long before the pandemic first surfaced in Wuhan, China in late 2019. The scheme was set into motion in mid-2019 with Big Tech clamping down on natural health websites in the guise of censoring what they claimed was "fake news." This was the first step in a master plan devised by Big Pharma and friends to force the majority of the world's population to turn to vaccines and medications to fight a perceived terrifying health threat, and in the process cash in on hundreds of billions in profits.

CENSORSHIP AND MEDIA CONTROL

In order for Big Pharma's plan to work, they needed to silence all voices that would see through the rouse and oppose them or offer more sensible solutions. That meant censoring natural health websites and blogs. If the population could not hear the truth, they would easily be led astray by the media, politicians, and health officials who are more than willing to act as Big Pharma's mouthpiece to spread fear and terror.

Big Pharma wields great influence and power among mainstream and social media, politicians, and health organizations worldwide. They have been cultivating relationships with these entities for years through advertising and donations, making these people and organizations dependent on the financial support of the drug industry. Have you noticed the hundreds of TV ads promoting drugs you've never heard of or will never need? Big Pharma doesn't spend millions of dollars in advertising each year simply to educate customers. Most of the drugs advertised are those that we cannot get without a doctor's prescription. After watching an advertisement, we don't rush out and buy the drug. These ads are not meant to influence us, they are meant as a means to control the media. With millions of dollars flowing into media outlets from the drug industry, editors and producers are well aware that any news they report that is uncomplimentary to the drug industry could be met with the threat of cutting off this huge inflow of adverting revenue.

The drug industry has been controlling most of the content in medical journals for years using this tactic. When editors have published studies criticizing certain drugs or that favor natural or inexpensive treatments over drugs, they have been threatened with the loss of Big Pharma advertising revenue. These journals often depend on drug company money to survive and consequently, capitulate and do whatever is necessary to placate Big Pharma.

This process has worked so well with the medical media that Big Pharma broadened its reach to mainstream media and social media as well. So much so, that they essentially control the vast majorly of the information we receive. In mid-2019 Big Pharma put their master plan of world subjection and mass vaccination into action by persuading Google, Facebook, Twitter, and other tech companies to censor natural health websites and voices. Google, for instance, revised how they manage their search rankings, giving preference to mainstream medical web pages that promote Big Pharma, such as Web MD, MedicineNet, and Wikipedia, while burying natural health websites so that they are extremely difficult if not impossible to find. Mercola.com which had been the number one natural health website on the internet and at the top of the list on Google searchers, suddenly dropped out of sight. Overnight, Mercola's website lost 90 percent of its internet traffic. The same thing occurred to all of the major natural websites. Google's reason for doing this was to censor what they considered to be "fake news." YouTube, which is owned by Google, began deleting videos promoting natural health solutions or that questioned the biased advice from mainstream media and those opposing Big Pharma's agenda. Facebook and others followed suit.[1]

Even Amazon.com censors books on COVID-19. When the paperback edition of this, *Plandemic*, was first submitted to Amazon.com, it was immediately banned. Essentially, I was told they would not allow it for sale because it did not conform to the information coming out of the WHO and the CDC, even though information from these organizations is often contradictory and continually changing. This book is listed on Amazon but it is permanently marked as "temporarily out of stock."

In order to stifle information about making informed decisions regarding the use of drugs and vaccines and to distort the benefits of natural approaches to healthcare, Big Pharma has employed an army of trolls to infiltrate social media. These trolls join natural health discussion groups and subscribe to online newsletters, posting comments on blogs and articles discreetly making their presence known by voicing opposing opinions that discredit natural solutions and promote the use of drugs. Big Pharma has done this for many years. These trolls have been particularly active during the COCID-19 crisis to oppose those who question the steps taken to manage the pandemic.

Some people may have doubts that Big Pharma really employs trolls. It sounds too much like a conspiracy theory. It's not. This fact is well known. In fact, the United Nations (UN) has publically come out and issued a call for volunteers to act as trolls to shut down opposition. In May 2020 the UN placed an open call for volunteers to help stop the spread of "misinformation." As a result, the UN has enlisted some 10,000 digital volunteers to go on social media platforms to promote the WHO's version of the pandemic and the need for drugs and vaccines before we can go back to normal. These volunteers receive daily emails instructing them how to counter opposing voices.[2]

Why would the UN be so involved in promoting the coronavirus pandemic? The WHO is an agency within the UN. The funding that comes to the WHO is also supporting the UN. Investigators at Devex found that as of June 30, 2020 the UN has received $471 million in funding to support their efforts to stamp out "misinformation" about the pandemic.[2]

DRACONIAN MEASURES INSTALLED

Within months after the initiation of the censorship a new virus appears in China, a virus that has never been seen before and one in which no one has had the opportunity to build an immunity to. A perfect virus for a worldwide pandemic that had the potential to cause as much destruction as the Spanish Flu Pandemic of 1918.

The virus seemed to come out of nowhere and rapidly spread from Wuhan, China to dozens of other counties in a matter of weeks, infecting thousands. The mainstream media immediately jumped in and began broadcasting dire warnings of a deadly pandemic encircling the globe, we were all in grave danger, they said. Nightly newscasters threw out the grim statistics of the number of new cases and deaths that occurred. The numbers were displayed daily as if they were reporting updates on the score of an ongoing championship game. It was like a game to them, each news outlet trying to outdo their competitors by reporting the most shocking statistics and predictions. It turned into a media frenzy of doom and gloom. Politicians and public health authorities sounded the alarm promoting the pandemic as a colossal health emergency. Scientists, using scanty data and computer models, predicted death rates in the millions and encouraged politicians to take drastic action. Instead of following traditional disease control measures that had been used in previous pandemics (such as quarantining the sick), massive lockdowns where hastily put into place to quarantine the healthy. Businesses, public services, parks, churches, and such were closed down and public gatherings forbidden. Only "essential" businesses and services were allowed to remain open. The politicians decided which were essential and which were not. People were divided into two classes: those who are considered "essential" and allowed to continue working, and those who were considered "nonessential" and barred from earning a living.

Small businesses and services judged to be "nonessential" were forced to close their doors while, paradoxically, everyone was free to roam through grocery stores, drug stores, and big box stores like Walmart, Target, and Home Depot, owned by big corporations. What we have allowed to be done in the name of public health has no parallel in history.

The world did not lock down during centuries of epidemics of smallpox, which was a highly contagious virus

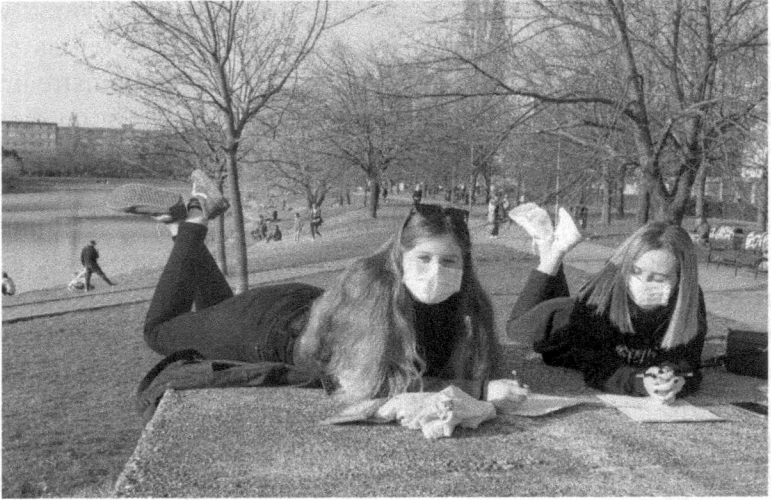

People were often required to wear face masks whenever they left their homes.

and had a case fatality rate of 30 percent. Societies have not closed businesses and schools to prevent tuberculosis, a contagious disease that spreads the same way as coronavirus and has a case fatality rate far higher than COVID-19.

News outlets, hospitals, big box stores, liquor stores, and marijuana dispensaries, were all pronounced essential services. While, daycare centers, natural health practitioners, dentists, family and mental health therapists, barbershops, and others were closed down. Even doctors and nurses who treat patients in need of non-urgent medical care and surgeries were deemed non-essential and forbidden to work, putting more than a million healthcare workers out of work in the US.[3] Most of the population was forbidden to go to work creating a great deal of unnecessary stress and anxiety, increasing the feelings of fear and panic.

Health officials claimed that the most dangerous people were not those that were obviously sick but those who were infected but did not show any symptoms. These were the most dangerous because they were unknowingly spreading the virus to others. For this reason, we were all told to wear masks and separate ourselves at least 6 feet apart from each other at all times, even outdoors. In New York City, residents were encouraged to take photos and report fellow citizens who violated social distancing rules by getting too close to each other outside. People were arrested for not wearing masks or for walking on deserted beaches, or for taking their children to empty playgrounds. Small business owners, struggling to feed their families, were sent to jail for reopening without government permission. In the meantime, prisons were releasing actual convicted criminals early in an effort to reduce the possible spread of the virus among inmates. Many of which were soon arrested again for violent assaults or other criminal activity.

Face masks have been recommended and even demanded everywhere. But do they work? Dr. Fauci insists we wear masks. In a CNN interview he assured us that he had all the answers by saying, "I think you can trust me" and other "experts." This is the same man that just a few months earlier stated on CBS News, "There's no reason to be walking around with a mask." Yet, other experts in public health dismissed surgical masks as inadequate protection from small airborne particles and warned that they did not form adequate seals around the face.

"Seriously people—stop buying masks!" said the US surgeon general, Dr. Jerome Adams. "They are not effective in preventing general public from catching coronavirus."

Dr. Michael Klompas and colleagues at Harvard Medical School and Brigham and Women's Hospital stated in a May article published in the *New England Journal of Medicine*, "We know that wearing a mask outside health care facilities offers little, if any, protection from infection...The chance of catching COVID-19 from a passing interaction in a public space is therefore minimal. In many cases, the desire for widespread masking is a reflexive reaction to anxiety over the pandemic."[4] Apparently, not everyone agrees with Fauci on the necessity of wearing masks, so which experts are we to believe?

Fauci tells us that we should believe the science. But what does the science say about face masks? After reviewing all of the published studies on the subject, Denis Rancourt, PhD, answered that question.[5] Rancourt states, "What I found when I looked at all the randomized controlled trials with verified outcome, meaning you actually measure whether or not the person was infected…NONE of these well-designed studies that are intended to remove observational bias… found there was a statistically significant advantage of wearing a mask versus not wearing a mask.

"We're talking many really [high-]quality trials. What this means—and this is very important—is that if there was any significant advantage to wearing a mask to reduce this [infection] risk, then you would have detected that in at least one of these trials, [yet] there's no sign of it.

"That to me is a firm scientific conclusion: There is no evidence that masks are of any utility either preventing the aerosol particles from coming out or from going in. You're not helping the people around you by wearing a mask, and you're not helping yourself preventing the disease by wearing a mask."

In spite of the drastic restrictions and regulations placed on us during the pandemic, they had virtually no effect. The virus ran its course regardless of the lockdowns and other measures taken to flatten the curve. According to a study by Professor Isaac Ben-Israel, chairman of the Israeli Space Agency and Council on Research and Development, "the spread of the coronavirus declines to almost zero after 70 days—no matter where it strikes, and no matter what measures governments impose to try to thwart it… Our analysis shows that this is a constant pattern across countries. Surprisingly, this pattern is common to countries that have taken a severe lockdown, including the paralysis of the economy, as well as to countries that implemented a far more lenient policy and have continued in ordinary life."[6]

STATISTICS ARE MANIPULATED

It is no secret the Big Pharma controls the actions of many politicians and government and private health officials. The World Health Organization is in the pocket of Big Pharma, as is the Centers for Disease Control and Prevention (CDC) and many others in the US, Europe, and elsewhere. These people and organizations receive funding and donations from Big Pharma, as well as their co-conspirator, the Bill and Melinda Gates Foundation. Like the media, this flow of cash influences what these organizations do and say. Under the control of their financial benefactors, they have been encouraged and even coached to blow this situation out of proportion and make it appear to be a far greater crisis than it really is.

An edict was sent out from the CDC to hospitals and healthcare providers across America instructing them to contribute deaths to COVID-19 regardless of the actual cause of death.[7] If the patient tested positive or even displayed any symptoms of a respiratory illness when they died, such as a fever or coughing which are also similar to the seasonal flu, then the death was attributed to COVID-19. People who were already suffering from terminal illness and in hospice or in the hospital and died from heart attacks, kidney failure, and cancer or even automobile accidents and suicide, if it was suspected they might have been infected with SARS-CoV-2, they became part of the death toll attributed to the virus.[8] In New York City, for example, funeral directors reported that doctors were putting COVID-19 as the cause of death on "everything." Regardless of the actual cause of death, they were all being reported as COVID-19 related.[9]

Health officials warned that if we relaxed the harsh isolation measures and allowed businesses to open and people to leave their homes, the number of cases of COVID-19 would rebound. As predicted, as the restrictions were loosed in June and July the number of COVID-19 cases made a dramatic jump. Were these numbers accurate? Apparently not. Although the number of people hospitalized increased, the death rate actually continued to decline. The vast majority of the people admitted to the hospital were not infected with the coronavirus but were the thousands of people who needed medical treatment months earlier but were forbidden or too frightened to go to the hospital during the peak of the outbreak. Once the restrictions were lifted they flooded into the hospitals to get much needed treatment for other conditions. Many of them were routinely tested for COVID-19. The number of positive results indicated a new surge in people coming down with COVID-19. The media was all over it, blaring out dire warnings of a resurgence of the disease.

However, COVID-19 death rates were declining. This is why the media never reported increasing death rates but only the number of cases. And even the number of cases reported were seriously wrong. The data was again being manipulated. This was revealed by investigators in Florida. In that state large numbers of COVID-19 cases were being reported as in many other locations. Looking at the numbers investigators found that some of the labs doing the testing were reporting nearly 100 percent positive cases—a total absurdity. Some of the labs were not reporting negative results at all. The investigators contacted every lab and found serious discrepancies with the state health departments reports. For example, Orlando Health was reported to have a 98 percent positivity rate, but hospital records indicated the rate was only 9.4 percent. The Orlando Veteran's Medical Center, which the health department said had a 76 percent rate, actually had only a 6 percent positivity rate.[10] That's why the death rates were so low, the actual cases were also declining.

This was obviously done to inflate the numbers so that greater fear could be projected. The data is being manipulated to match the dire projections predicted by the computer models. We cannot trust the statistics thrust at us by the media.

6

Are Drugs and Vaccines the Answer?

SOLUTIONS THAT WORK ARE BEING IGNORED, CENSORED, AND ATTACKED

Never has there been a time in history where health information has been so aggressively censored and in some cases attacked. Only one viewpoint is allowed. All talk about potentially beneficial natural or alternative solutions are forbidden. Even discussions about harmless measures, like taking vitamin supplements, are banned or ridiculed.

Vitamin D has been shown to boost the immune system and be an effective weapon against coronaviruses.[1-2] At the beginning of the pandemic I watched a YouTube video produced by a medical doctor explaining how vitamin D could stop SARS-CoV-2. She explained in detail how the vitamin worked to inactivate the virus and cited over a dozen studies, backing up every statement with published research. Two months later I went back to view the video again, but found that Google had deleted it as part of their so-called "false news" censorship campaign. Many other YouTube videos from scientists and physicians, even those with top-tier credentials, were deleted in a universal attempt to censor all natural solutions that may have great potential to save hundreds of thousands of lives, ease people's fears, and give them hope.

Simply exposing 40 percent of our skin to direct sunlight for 15 to 30 minutes a day can give us substantial resistance to COVID-19. Vitamin D is produced in the skin from the ultraviolet (UV) rays from the sun. Vitamin D has an incredible ability to boost the effectiveness of the immune system and protect us from viral infections.[3] This is why viruses, such as colds and flu are seasonal. They are most prominent during the winter months when people spend most of their time indoors, and decline in the spring and summer as people get outdoors and increase their sun exposure. This is a very simple and cost-free strategy to prevent viral infections, including COVID-19.

Low blood levels of vitamin D makes you more susceptible to infection by the coronavirus and studies have shown that people with COVID-19 have low vitamin D levels.[4] Studies have also shown that as vitamin D levels increase, deaths from COVID-19 decline.[5]

This pattern is clearly evident in the European population, see the graph on the followng page. A comparison of COVID-19 deaths with blood vitamin D levels shows the declining deaths with increasing vitamin D levels. Italy and Spain were especially hit hard by COVID-19 and have among the lowest vitamin D levels. The elderly generally have lower vitamin D levels making them more vulnerable to the coronavirus. As seen in the graph, the elderly in both countries had the highest percentage of deaths.[6]

When sun exposure isn't feasible, you can take dietary supplements. Most government recommendations for vitamin D intake range from 400 to 600 IU per day. These values are based on what is required for bone health but are not adequate for protection against COVID-19. Adults need to take about 4,000 IU per day to achieved the blood levels found to protect against the coronavirus.[7]

Vitamin C has also been recommended and in some hospitals is being used to treat patients with COVID-19. Studies are currently underway to confirm the effectiveness of high-dose vitamin C in treating this infection.[8] Quercetin, deaths/1M population

25(OH)D mean nmol/L

350 — 300 — 250 — 200 — 150 — 100 — 50 — 0

0 — 10 — 20 — 30 — 40 — 50 — 60 — 70 — 80 — 90 — 100

Spain older
Italy older
Italy
Spain
Belgium
France
Netherlands
Switzerland
UK
Sweden
Ireland
Denmark
Germany
Iceland
Norway
Portugal
Estonia
Turkey
Hungary
Finland
Slovakia

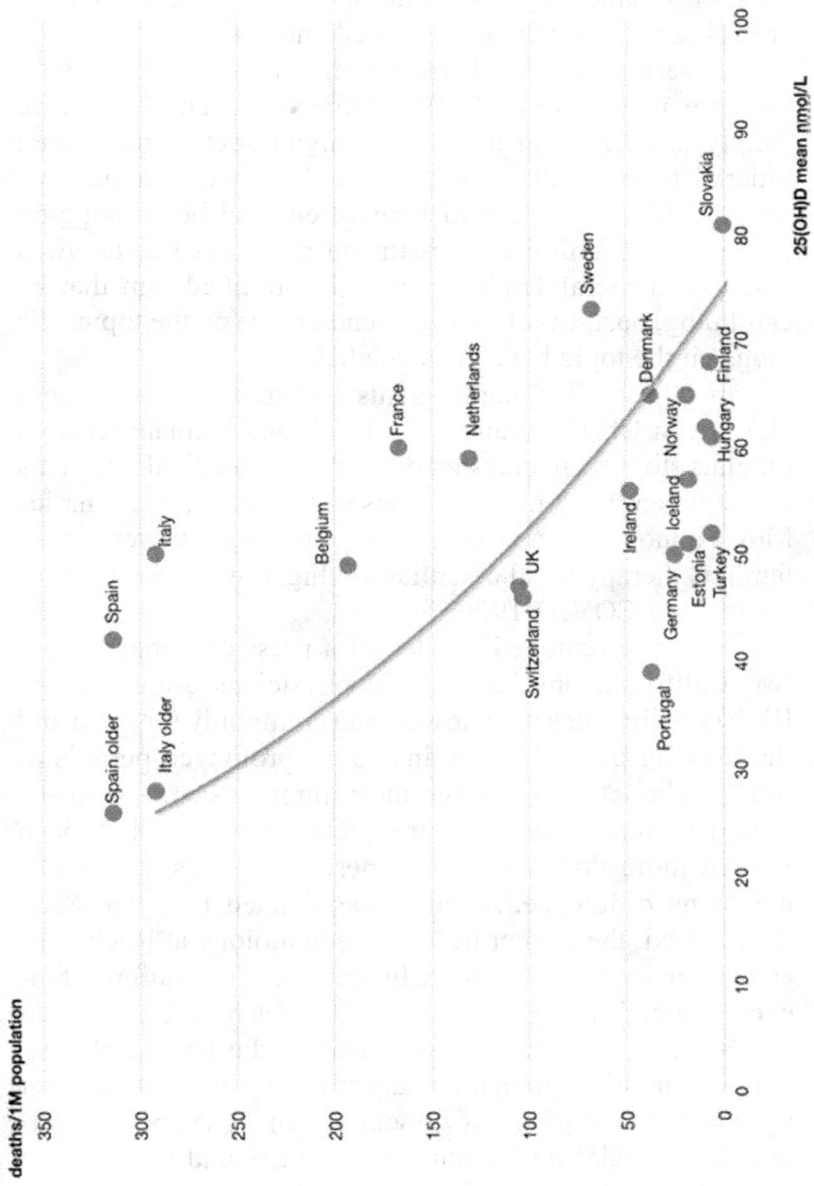

zinc, and molecular hydrogen have also been recommended as possible means to fight the coronavirus.[9-10] In the meantime, information about vitamins and other natural therapies are being aggressively discouraged and censored.

Government officials have been targeting doctors who promote natural COVID-19 treatments, even if they are simply talking about it. Two Michigan doctors have been ordered to stop talking about or using natural treatments for COVID-19. Dr. David Brownstein had been blogging on various vitamin-based treatment protocols for the virus when the Federal Trade Commission notified him that he can't blog, post, tweet, or even send emails on the topic. His blogs on the topic have been deleted.

In late April, federal agents outfitted in tactical gear along with US Department of Health and Human Services officials stormed in and shut down Allure Medical Spa. This was apparently done in response to founder, Dr. Charles Mok's announcement that he was providing intravenous vitamin C therapy to all essential Michigan workers at risk of contracting COVID-19.[11]

YouTube removed a video of a press conference from two California physicians. The physicians argued COVID-19 fatality rates were lower than commonly reported and that forcing people to stay inside for prolonged periods of time might actually damage their immune systems. At the time YouTube removed it, the press conference had been viewed more than 5 million times. A person's credentials makes no difference. A video was deleted from Dr. Knut Wittkowski, the former head of epidemiology at Rockefeller University's Center for Clinical and Translational Science, criticizing lockdowns. The list goes on and on.

Social media giants have become the unofficial marketing arm of Big Pharma, aggressively promoting their agenda and censoring any dissenting voices. As private corporations, social media outlets are not bound by the First Amendment (freedom of speech) and can block any communication they desire.

The lockdowns have been a clever pre-planned strategy to isolate people from one another and prevent the sharing of ideas and solutions that may challenge the current status quo. Without the option to gather in groups, information must be disseminated by social media. However, censorship by Facebook, Twitter, YouTube, and others has prevented this exchange of knowledge and ideas.

When people started to complain about censorship, Susan Wojcicki, the chief executive of YouTube, told CNN that YouTube would ban all videos contradicting World Health Organization statements and guidelines about coronavirus, including the stay at home messages and the wearing of masks.

The leadership of the WHO is controlled by the Bill and Melinda Gates Foundation and for this reason is highly biased. Sometimes truthful information from honest scientists working for WHO is published online and then later rescinded and revised. Consequently, the information they have been disseminating about the pandemic has been contradictory and often erroneous.[12] For example, stating that antibodies to coronavirus do not confer immunity to the virus, then hours later deleting that message and reporting antibodies likely "provide some level of protection." On April 6, 2020, the WHO publicly released guidance saying that healthy people do not need to wear face masks and that doing so won't provide any added protection from the coronavirus.[13] Then on June 5, they reversed their statement saying everyone needed to wear masks. Wojcicki didn't mention how YouTube might treat these spontaneous reversals in WHO messaging.

Meanwhile, Facebook, which is used by more than half of all Americans, has repeatedly censored groups trying to organize anti-lockdown protests. "Events that defy governments' guidance on social distancing aren't allowed on Facebook," a Facebook spokesman said. On May 13, Facebook took its most aggressive action yet, removing the

380,000-member group "Michiganders Against Excessive Quarantine," one of the original anti-lockdown groups. It then quickly removed a replacement group called "Stand Up Michigan." When it comes to voicing opinions about the coronavirus, there is clearly no freedom of speech on social media.

Even cheap generic medications, such as the malaria drug hydroxychloroquine, are denounced as dangerous and information about them censored. Hydroxychloroquine, a drug that has been in use for some 60 years, was found to be effective against the coronavirus. This isn't a new discovery. Studies as far back as 2005 demonstrated its antiviral effect against SARS-CoV, the older cousin to SARS-CoV-2. So, it was logical to assume it might also be useful during the current pandemic, especially when combined with zinc.[14-15] And it has been. Early studies in France and clinical outcomes from multiple treating physicians using the drug provided hope to combat the virus. In addition to combating coronaviruses, it has also found use in the treatment of arthritis, lupus, diabetes, and cancer.[16-17]

The patent on this drug expired years ago, making it very inexpensive and widely available. It has been used for decades and considered safe all that time, but suddenly it is deemed too dangerous. We were warned not to used it as it might cause heart arrhythmia. Studies were quickly done to evaluate the drug for the treatment of COVID-19 and the results showed it to be worthless and even dangerous.

Why are they going after this drug so aggressively? Perhaps because it provides a cheap solution so that there would be no need for newly patented and expensive antivirals or new vaccines? That would put a deep dent in the profits anticipated by Big Pharma, so they have to attack it and discourage its use. Despite the testimony of many doctors who are using the drug with great success and with little adverse effects, the drug is heavily criticized. Within a short period a time, a study was published that claimed hydroxychloroquine did not work and was dangerous, just as the Big Pharma puppets had been saying. However, the study was riddled with inconsistencies which were plainly evident causing a outcry from physicians to reexamine the data. At first, the authors of the study refused to share their data, but under pressure they admitted they didn't have all the data. The company the authors used to analyze the data, refused to cooperate or release the information to independent reviewers. It appeared they had used bogus data. To save face, the authors retracted two studies, one published in the *Lancet* and the other in *The New England Journal of Medicine*.[18]

Several other studies were also published that concluded that hydroxychloroquine was ineffective against COVID-19. However when you examine the data in these studies you find that they used very high, toxic doses of the drug and administered it to patients who were already well advanced with the disease. It is strange that critics of hydroxychloroquine claim that the drug is too toxic to treat COVID-19, yet in these studies they used doses far above that which is recommended. Also, like most antivirals, hydroxychloroquine is most effective when treatment is started as early as possible. As the infection progresses, it is much harder to treat. But in these studies the disease was always advanced. In addition, none of these studies included zinc. Hydroxychloroquine's antiviral effects are enhanced when combined with zinc. The drug acts as a key that opens the door on the cell membrane allowing zinc to enter. Zinc keeps the virus from replicating. These studies were funded by the Bill and Melinda Gates Foundation, WHO, and others—organizations that have a vested interest and don't want the drug to be used to treat COVID-19.

It appears these studies were designed to guarantee the drug would be a failure and even produce adverse effects. These studies were widely quoted as proof that hydroxychloroquine was useless and possibly dangerous. They were used as marketing tools to promote false information. Hmmm...fake news from the Big Pharma controlled medical media. This should sound alarm bells as to who is really giving us the fake health news.

Following on the tail of these flawed studies a new, high-quality study by researchers from the Henry Ford Health System was released. The study reported that treatment with hydroxychloroquine significantly cuts the death rate of sick hospitalized patients suffering from COVID-19. The large-scale study analyzed 2,541 patients hospitalized between March 10 and May 2, 2020 across the system's six hospitals. The study found 13 percent of those treated with hydroxychloroquine alone died, compared to 26.4 percent not treated with hydroxychloroquine. The drug cut the fatality rate by half. This study came directly from examining real people with actual diagnoses under medical supervision, not some mysterious databank of questionable reliability. No adverse effects of any consequence were reported.

"Our analysis shows that using hydroxychloroquine helped saves lives," said neurosurgeon Dr. Steven Kalkanis, CEO, Henry Ford Medical Group and Senior Vice President and Chief Academic Officer of Henry Ford Health System. "As doctors and scientists, we look to the data for insight. And the data here is clear that there was benefit to using the drug as a treatment for sick, hospitalized patients."[19]

French science-prize winning microbiologist and infectious disease expert Didier Raoult, founder and director of the research hospital Institut Hospitalo-Universitaire Méditerranée Infection, reported that a combination of hydroxychloroquine and azithromycin (an antibiotic to treat secondary infections), administered immediately upon diagnosis, led to recovery and the absence of the coronavirus in nasal swabs in 91.7 percent of patients.[20]

Dr. Vladimir Zelenko reports that a combination of hydroxychloroquine, azithromycin, and zinc sulfate given for 5 days has lead to a near 100 percent recovery rate of COVID-19 when given within 5 days of the onset of symptoms. In a clinical study, Zelenko showed that among those patients receiving the triple combination of hydroxychloroquine, azithromycin, and zinc, there were 5 times fewer deaths in comparison to those receiving conventional treatment.[21] Zelenko contends that doctors and public health administrators who discourage the use of hydroxychloroquine and prevent patients from getting this treatment are guilty of mass murder. Positive information about hydroxychloroquine is actively being censored. A group of physicians who have been successfully using the drug posted footage of their experiences and success. As soon as their pro-hydroxychloroquine statements went viral, Facebook, YouTube, and Twitter immediately blocked it. Fake news, they claim.

The physicians, who call themselves "America's Frontline Doctors," had a website that went dark after the social media monopoly censored their video. Visitors to the site see a message that says "website expired."

Depriving these doctors the right to share their medical observations and opinions was not allowed by those who control social media, nor have their voices been allowed in mainstream media either. If erasing their video and website were not enough, trolls hiding on discussion groups and social media came out in full force to denounce the physicians as quacks or shysters trying to make a quick buck. They even attacked the physician's personal and religious beliefs in an attempt to discredit them.

Members of America's Frontline Doctors are not the only physicians who champion hydroxychloroquine as a COVID-19 treatment. Physicians all over the country are quietly prescribing it to their patients, friends, and family members. Among them is Dr. Harvey Risch, a medical doctor and professor epidemiology at the Yale School of Public Health. Dr. Risch has written more than 300 peer-reviewed medical articles and holds senior positions on the editorial boards of several leading medical journals. Who do you believe? Do you believe Dr. Risch and his fellow physicians who have firsthand experience treating COVID-19 patients? Or, do you believe the owners of Facebook, Google, and Twitter and the journalists at CNN and the New York Times, who haven't spent a day in medical school?

"Tens of thousands of patients with COVID-19 are dying unnecessarily. Fortunately, the situation can be reversed easily and quickly," Dr. Risch wrote in *Newsweek*, on July 23, 2020. "I am referring of course, to the medication hydroxychloroquine. When this inexpensive oral medication is given very early in the course of illness…it has shown to be highly effective, especially when given in combination with the antibiotics azithromycin or doxycycline and the nutritional supplement zinc." Dr Risch went on and described 8 peer-reviewed studies that attest to the efficacy of hydroxychloroquine in treating COVID-19. Yet, voices promoting the use of the drug have been censored. In some jurisdictions, doctors have even been banned from prescribing the drug.

"I myself know of 2 doctors who have saved the lives of hundreds of patients with these medications, but are now fighting state medical boards to save their licenses and reputations," Dr. Risch wrote. "The cases against them are completely without scientific merit."

Just like Dr. Li Wenliang in Wuhan, who was reprimanded and censored for spreading "rumors" about the impending pandemic, doctors in the US are being punished and censored for spreading "rumors," or as the media calls it, "fake news."

Public health officials and governmental authorities are actively discouraging the use of any currently available (and inexpensive) therapy that might help. In the absence of a vaccine or any other drug-based therapy, anything that might help would be of great benefit. Yet, there is a highly aggressive movement to prevent any treatment of COVID-19 until new (and expensive) drugs become available.

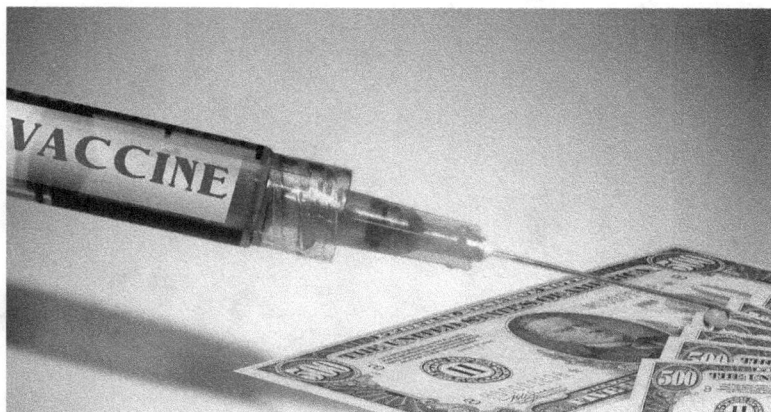

DRUGS AND VACCINES ARE PROMOTED
AS THE ONLY SOLUTION

Health officials and politicians insist that only newly developed (meaning protected by patent and expensive) antivirals and vaccines can stop the virus. They say we currently have nothing to fight it with (more fake news). Vaccine makers have been given the green light to fast-track vaccines and make them available worldwide. Politicians hinted at the possibility of forced vaccinations. Children would need them to go back to school. Healthcare workers and first responders would need them to work. Everyone would be tracked and tagged to identify if they have had the virus and if they had been vaccinated. Vaccination would be mandatory for all.

Dr. Anthony Fauci, director of the NIAID, has been the face of the coronavirus taskforce in the US since the beginning of the pandemic. He insists that we stay locked down and continue social distancing until a vaccine is made available and everyone has been vaccinated. Then the country can be opened up again.

There are currently more than 100 research programs around the world working on developing COVID-19 vac-

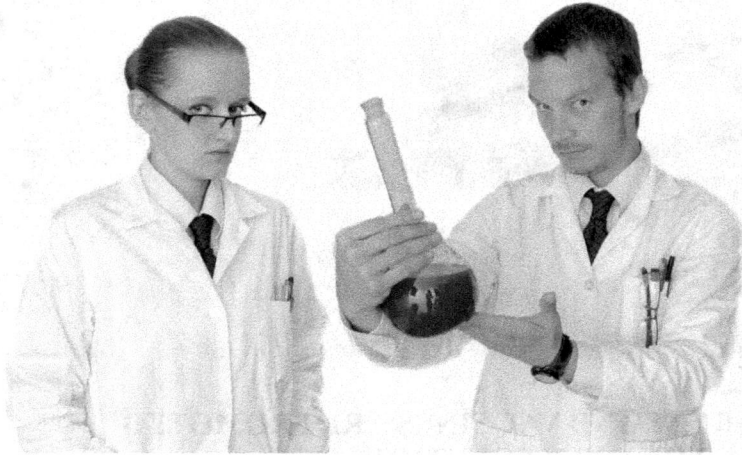

Drugs and vaccines are being fast-tracked into production to firght COVID-19.

cines, including 10 that have reached the clinical evaluation stage as of June 2020. Fast-tracking allows them to skip important steps, such as adequate animal testing, to assure safety. Fast-tracking, allows developers to skip some of the testing procedures and go straight to human trials. If no serious side effects occur after a few of weeks, the vaccine is considered safe and can be mass produced and distributed. One problem is that serious side effects may not show up until several months later.

On March 16, 2020, Moderna was the first company to begin human testing of a COVID-19 vaccine. The trial involved 45 healthy adults between the ages of 18 and 55. Six weeks later, the company announced the trial a resounding success, despite the fact that only 8 of the participants developed any antibodies to the virus and more than half experienced adverse reactions that included fatigue, chills, headache, fever, myalgia, and lingering injection site pain. The reactions in 3 of the participants were serious enough to require medical intervention. Keep in mind, this was among volunteers who were healthy and had no known health problems—the type of individuals who are not seriously affected by the coronavirus. If the vaccine were administered to those who would need protection from the virus the most—those who do have underlying health problems—the vaccine could prove far more dangerous. Out of the 45 participants, 37 showed no benefit, which makes you wonder how these results could be considered a success. The treatment would likely require repeated vaccinations to increase the likelihood of generating antibodies, but also increase the risk of adverse reactions. If the vaccine were to be approved and given to millions of people it would cause far more harm than the virus itself.

Moderna did not explain why it reported positive antibody tests for only 8 of the participants. It also suspiciously failed to report any data from mouse studies. Fauci had waved ferret and primate studies to allow Moderna to fast-track the vaccine to human trials.

One of Moderna's volunteers, Ian Haydon, 29, of Seattle has spoken out about the severe adverse reactions he suffered 12 hours after receiving the second of two doses of the vaccine. Hayden is one of the 4 participants who had serious reactions and one of three who experienced Grade 3 "systemic symptoms" requiring medical intervention.

According to William Schaffner, MD, professor of preventive medicine and infectious diseases at Vanderbilt University Medical Center, Haydon's reactions to the vaccine are "noteworthy," but that it doesn't "stop the train," suggesting research and development of Moderna's vaccine would continue full speed ahead.[22]

Try as one might to downplay Haydon's adverse reactions and those of the other participants in Moderna's trial, these were severe reactions. What is noteworthy is that 9 percent of the participants experienced these reactions. If just 1 million people received the vaccine, 90,000 people would suffer a serious adverse reaction. Imagine what this would mean were this vaccine to be given to tens of millions of people?

Since this trial was pronounced a success, it may be among the first COVID-19 vaccines put into mass production. If other vaccines are of equal effectiveness, mass vaccinations will produce devastating results.

CanSino Biologies, Inc. of Tianjin, China, in partnership with China's Academy of Military Medical Sciences' Institute of Biotechnology has been testing another COVID-19 vaccine. Their first trial involved 108 participants ranging from 45 to 60 years of age. After the first phase, 87 (83 percent) of the participants suffered at least one adverse reaction within 7 days after vaccination. Since the exact amount of the vaccine needed was not yet determined, the subjects were separated into 3 groups: high, medium, and low dose. Overall, 9 percent of the participants experienced Grade 3 adverse reactions. Of the 36 participants in the high dose group, 17 percent of them had Grade 3 reactions, which required medical intervention.

The most common adverse reaction was abnormal pain at the injection site, which was reported in 54 percent vaccine recipients. Pain was reported in 47 percent participants in the low dose group, 56 percent participants in the middle dose group, and 58 percent participants in the high dose group. The most commonly reported systematic adverse reactions overall were fever (46 percent), fatigue (44 percent), headache (39 percent), and muscle pain (17 percent). Fever was reported in 42 percent of the participants in the low dose group, 42 percent of the participants in the middle dose group, and 56 percent of the participants in the high dose group. Headache was reported in 39 percent of the participants in the low dose group, 31 percent of the participants in the middle dose group, and 47 percent of the participants in the high dose group. Muscle pain was reported in 19 percent of the participants in the low dose group, 8 percent of the participants in the middle dose group, and 22 percent of the participants in the high dose group.[23]

Despite the adverse effects, the excuse to justify the use of these vaccines is that they may save lives. Sure there may be some collateral damage, some people will get gravely sick, some may even die, but for the greater good of everybody the risk is worth the price. However, what if you or a family member is among those who suffer severe and possibly permanent damage, is it worth the price?

Past attempts at developing coronavirus vaccines have always failed. Coronavirus vaccine development began after the SARS outbreak in 2002. About 30 vaccines were developed. The most promising vaccines were administered to ferrets, which produced a robust antibody response, indicating their bodies were capable of fighting off the infection. However, when the ferrets were then exposed to the wild virus, they developed inflammation in all of their organs, their lungs stopped functioning, and they died.[24] The vaccine made an infection from the actual virus far more deadly.

Dr. Fauci has expressed uncertainty about the length of protection a successful COVID-19 vaccine would provide. It may raise antibodies for only a few months or for as long as a year. Booster shots may be needed a few months later.[25] All of the front-line vaccine developers are aiming for a two-shot administration. It may also turn into an annual vaccine like the flu shot. Although children are rarely infected by COVID-19 it may become part of the suite of vaccinations mandated as part of the childhood immunization schedule. If a COVID-19 vaccine proves successful, or at least minimally harmful, it has the potential to generate billions in profits for the developers.

REMDESIVIR

Gilead Sciences is the maker of remdesivir, the first antiviral drug recommended by the WHO to treat COVID-19.

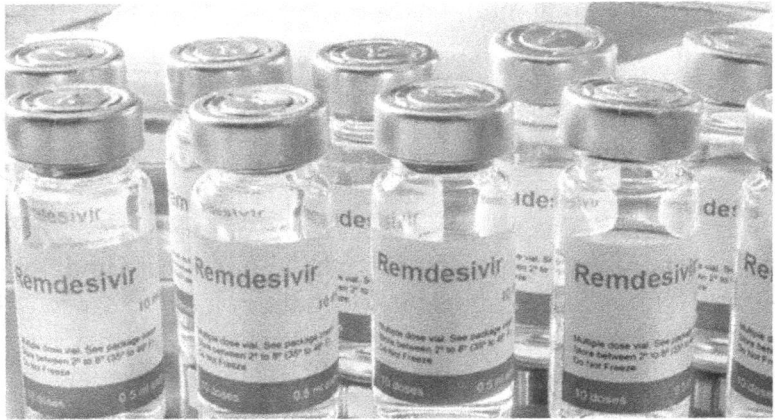

It was not originally meant to treat the coronavirus but was developed to fight other viruses, in particular Ebola. However, it was shown to be ineffective and up until 2020 had not been approved to treat anything. At the onset of the CO-VID-19 pandemic, drug companies began looking at their current inventory of drugs to see if anything they already had on the shelf might be useful in fighting the coronavirus. Gilead's remdesivir, which had been sitting in limbo since its disappointing performance against other viruses, was immediately resurrected as a possible candidate.

The first study published to evaluate remdesivir's effect on COVID-19 came out in April 2020. The randomized, double-blind, placebo-controlled study involved 237 hospitalized patients found no statistical difference between remdesivir and a placebo.[26] This was a hard blow to Gilead, but two more studies were in the works.

In a second study, clinical improvement was observed in 36 of 53 hospital patients (68 percent) that received remdesivir.[27] However, this study did not include a control group for comparison. Simply taking a medicine can have a placebo effect in which patients can improve even though the drug may have no real effect. Although promising, the results were inconclusive.

In the third study, remdesivir was shown to shorten recovery time for hospitalized patients with COVID-19, although it had essentially no impact on reducing the risk of death.[28] This study was conducted by scientists from the National Institute of Allergy and Infectious Diseases, the organization headed by Anthony Fauci. When the study was released, Fauci enthusiastically promoted remdesivir as a potential "game-changer" and stated that the drug could become the "standard of care" for COVID-19.

The editors of the *British Medical Journal* (BMJ) questioned the financial links and bias in the third study. Twelve percent of the participants taking remdesivir stopped treatment early because of adverse effects, compared to 5 percent of the placebo group. The trial was stopped before meeting recruitment targets, so results were inconclusive but did not rule out the possibility of benefit. The editors of the BMJ described the study results as "lackluster."[29] One of the study's investigators was a Gilead employee and six other authors declared financial ties to Gilead. In addition, representatives from Gilead participated in the protocol development and in weekly protocol team discussions—a level of engagement suggesting this drug trial could not be regarded as independent from the manufacturer and, therefore, was highly likely to show bias. Midway through the trial the primary outcome was changed from the number of deaths to the number of people reportedly feeling better, apparently because the desired results were not favorable. In addition, participants were allowed to switch from the placebo to remdesivir, bringing an early end to masking for some participants affecting the outcome. Consequently, the study could not claim to be double-blind and was subject to bias. Despite these shenanigans and ignoring the dismal results from the first study that was double-blinded and randomized, with the hearty endorsement of Dr. Fauci, the FDA approved the drug for the treatment of COVID-19.

Interestingly, as soon as remdesivir was put into use to treat COVID-19, serious problems quickly surfaced—multiple cases of liver damage were being reported by physicians.[30] A case study published soon after the approval of the drug found that out of 5 patients with COVID-19, 4 of them had to stop treatment due to liver and kidney damage. Two of the patients suffered kidney failure—a life threatening condition.[31] That is one of the problems of hastily approving a drug to treat a health crisis, serious adverse reactions are not always recognized at first. Remdesivir's hasty approval based on questionable evidence of its effectiveness and total lack of investigation on its safety, allowed a drug of questionable worth and the potential to do great harm to be distributed globally.

The drugs and vaccines developed without the requirements for all the normal safety testing, may cause untold injuries and deaths, but the drug companies are not concerned. They will not be held responsible for any injury caused by these products. Under the Pandemic and All Hazards Preparedness Act passed by the US Congress in December 2006, pharmaceutical companies are immune to all civil liability from injuries and deaths caused by vaccines and drugs manufactured in response to a declared public health emergency. Any drugs developed in response to the COVID-19 pandemic fits into that category, no matter what harm these drugs may cause, people cannot get compensation from the drug makers. We use these drugs at our own risk. For this reason, it is wise to investigate the side effects and effectiveness of any drug before receiving it. Don't take your doctor's word that a drug is safe, if it was properly prescribed and you suffer a crippling reaction, you can't get compensation from the doctor or drug maker.

7

Who is Behind the Pandemic?

BILL GATES PLANS TO VACCINATE THE WORLD

"Until we get almost everybody vaccinated globally, we still won't be back to normal," declared Bill Gates.[1] Does that mean we must continue to distance ourselves from others, be required to wear masks, and limit activity outside our homes until there is a vaccine available and administered to all? If Bill Gates has his way, yes.

Bill Gates is no public health expert. He is not a doctor, an epidemiologist, or an infectious disease researcher. Yet, somehow he has become a central figure in the lives of billions of people, presuming to dictate the medical actions that will be required for the world to go "back to normal." The transformation of Bill Gates from computer kingpin to global health czar tells us a great deal about where we are heading as the world struggles with a mostly manufactured health crisis.

Bill Gates has spent much of the past two decades transforming himself from software billionaire into a benefactor of humanity through his Bill & Melinda Gates Foundation. With $46.8 billion in assets on its books, the Bill & Melinda Gates Foundation wields enormous power and influence over global health policy.

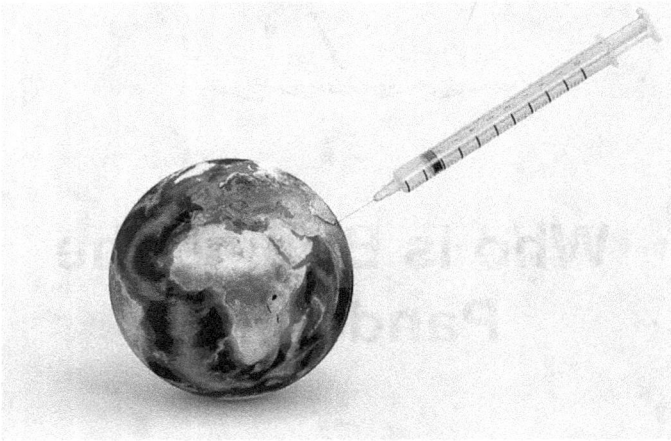

The Bill & Melinda Gates Foundation spends tens of millions of dollars each year on media partnerships, sponsoring coverage of its program areas across the board. Gates funds The Guardian's Global Development website, NPR's global health coverage, and the Our World in Data website that tracks the latest statistics and research on the coronavirus pandemic. Gates funds BBC coverage of global health and development issues, both through its BBC Media Action organization and the BBC itself. Gates also funds world health coverage on ABC News.

When the PBS's NewsHour with Jim Lehrer was given a $3.5 million Gates Foundation grant to set up a special unit to report on global health issues, NewsHour communications chief Rob Flynn was asked about the potential conflict of interest that it would have in reporting on issues that the Gates Foundation is itself involved in. "In some regards I guess you might say that there are not a heck of a lot of things you could touch in global health these days that would not have some kind of Gates tentacle," Flynn responded.[2] Indeed, it would be almost impossible to find any area of global health that has been left untouched by the tentacles of the Bill & Melinda Gates Foundation.

It was Gates who sponsored the meeting that led to the creation of Gavi, the Vaccine Alliance, a global public-private partnership bringing together state sponsors and big pharmaceutical companies, whose specific goals include the creation of "healthy markets for vaccines and other immunization products."[3] As a founding partner of the alliance, the Gates Foundation provided $750 million in seed funding and has gone on to make over $4.1 billion in commitments to the group.

When a public-private partnership of governments, world health bodies, and 13 leading pharmaceutical companies came together in 2012 "to accelerate progress toward eliminating or controlling 10 neglected tropical diseases," there was the Gates Foundation with $363 million of support.[4]

When the Coalition for Epidemic Preparedness Innovations was launched at the World Economic Forum in Davos in 2017 to develop vaccines against emerging infectious diseases, there was the Gates Foundation with an initial injection of $100 million.[5]

The Bill & Melinda Gates Foundation's fingerprints can be seen on every major global health initiative of the past two decades. It comes as no surprise, then, that—far beyond the $250 million that the Gates Foundation has pledged to the "fight" against coronavirus—every aspect of the current coronavirus pandemic involves organizations, groups and individuals with direct ties to Gates funding.[6]

From the start, the World Health Organization has been the body setting the guidelines and recommendations shaping the global response to this outbreak. The organization is largely reliant on funds from the Bill & Melinda Gates Foundation. The WHO's most recent donor report shows that the Bill & Melinda Gates Foundation is the organization's second-largest donor behind the United States government.[7] The Gates Foundation single-handedly contributes more to the world health body than Australia, Canada, France, Germany, Russia and the UK combined.

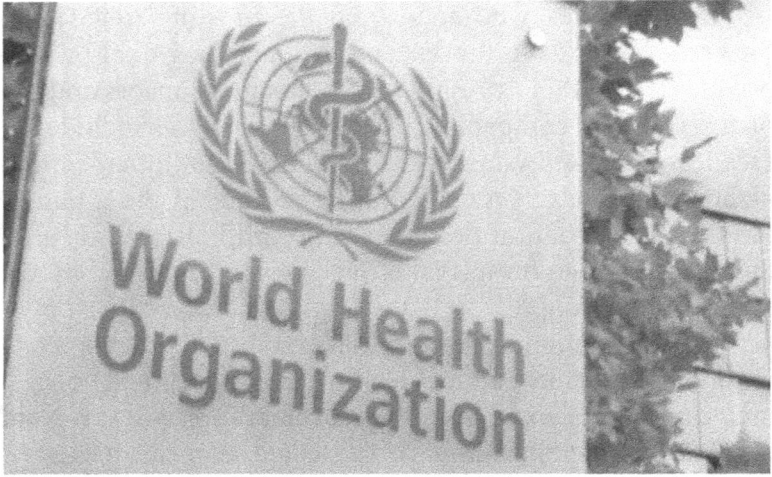

What's more, current World Health Organization Director-General, Tedros Adhanom Ghebreyesus, like Bill Gates himself, is not a medical doctor at all, but the controversial ex-Minister of Health of Ethiopia, who was accused of covering up three cholera outbreaks in the country during his tenure.[8] Before joining the WHO, he sat on the board of the Gates-founded Gavi, the Vaccine Alliance, and the other Gates-funded organizations. He has now been accused of mismanaging the current coronavirus pandemic, making it far worse globally because of his initial inaction and assurance that China had things under control and that there was nothing for us to worry about.

Bill Gates' ultimate goal is to vaccinate the world by any means possible. Why is Gates so interested in our welfare? Is he really that concerned about you? What do people normally do who have billions of dollars of surplus money lying around? They invest it to produce even more money. This investment goes to highly profitable corporations. Among the most profitable corporations in the world are those in the pharmaceutical and healthcare industry. As their profits go up, their investors get richer. Vaccines are a huge cash cow for drug makers. The Bill & Melisa Gates

Foundation owns hundreds of millions of dollars in stocks and bonds in drug companies.[9] At least 10 vaccine makers including, GlaxoSmithKline, Johnson & Johnson, Roche, Pfizer, Merck, Novartis, and Sanofi, all of which are working on COVID-19 vaccines, have direct ties to the Bill & Melinda Gates Foundation.

The Bill & Melinda Gates Foundation is a major source of funding for WHO, CDC, and the National Institutes of Health (NIH), all of which are the primary forces driving public policy that involves the draconian lockdowns and social distancing measures we are experiencing. Gates is also the source for Microsoft's ambition to establish a global vaccination ID program, in which everyone's vaccination history will be recorded and made available to government officials, potential employers, school admissions, and others and to track those who have not received all mandated vaccinations.

PANDEMIC PROFITEERS

If you want to know who is at the bottom of this pandemic, all you need to do is follow the money. Who is profiting the most from this crisis? Could they have had any influence over how the crisis has been handled? Could they have even been involved from the start? Considering some of the insane measures taken during the crisis, it becomes obvious it isn't all about public health, it is about power and greed.

As a result of the stay-at-home orders and business closures, millions of people were left jobless. Many small businesses couldn't survive and shut down permanently. Others struggled under harsh restrictions that limited their ability to operate at full capacity. Unemployment was at its highest since the Great Depression. Forty million Americans were out of work. The situation was much the same in other countries.

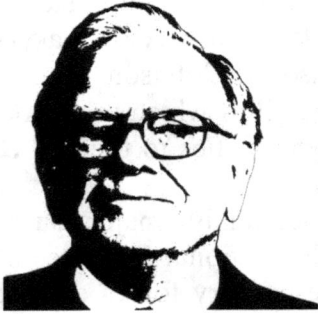

Widespread fear is your friend as an investor because it serves up bargain purchases.

Warren Buffett

The COVID-19 pandemic ignited global fear causing the stock market to crash. Warren Buffett, chairman of the holding company Berkshire Hathaway, and one of the richest men in the world stated, "Widespread fear is your friend as an investor because it serves up bargain purchases." MoneyTalks-News, December 30, 2018.

A report by the Well Being Trust and the Robert Graham Center for Policy Studies in Family Medicine and Primary Care indicates that as many as 75,000 Americans may have died from the COVID-19 pandemic due to drug or alcohol misuse and suicide, which they attribute to "deaths of despair." These deaths were not caused by the virus, but by media fearmongering, forced self-isolation, unprecedented economic failure, and massive unemployment.[10]

While most people's lives have been upended and many suffered financial hardships, not everyone, however, suffered from unemployment, isolation, fear, and despair as the rest of us have. Some of the richest people in the world who control the healthcare and biotech industries, are profiting handsomely from the COVID-19 pandemic.

As millions worldwide suffered financial crises, billionaires everywhere were reaping a fortune. According to the Institute for Policy Studies (IPS), as of June 18, 2020 US billionaire wealth increased by $584 billion, since the start of the pandemic. At least 29 new billionaires joined the ranks among the richest Americans. From January 1,

2020 to April 10, 2020, the wealth of 34 of the richest billionaires increased by tens of millions of dollars and 8 had their net worth rise by more than $1 billion.[11] The top five billionaires—Jeff Bezos (Amazon's CEO), Bill Gates, Mark Zuckerberg (Facebook's CEO), Warren Buffett (who contributed $31 billion to help fund the Gates Foundation), and Larry Ellison—saw their wealth grow by a total of $101.7 billion.[12] These people own hundreds of thousands of shares of stocks in numerous drug and biotech companies. The increase in value of these companies during the pandemic has boosted their fortunes by tens of billions of dollars. Bill Gates' campaign to vaccinate the world has greatly enriched himself and the other members of the billionaires club.

Responding to the urging by public health officials and drug company lobbyists, the US Congress passed the CARES Act signed into law on Mar. 27, 2020 that will cost American taxpayers over two trillion dollars. The federal legislation includes $27 billion for development of COVID-19 vaccines, drug therapies, and the purchase of pandemic medical supplies like face masks, ventilators, and testing kits. The legislation did not include a cap placed on how much money drug companies can charge and profits they can make on the COVID-19 vaccines and drug therapies they develop with the use of taxpayer money they received for free from the government.

On March 30, just three days after the CARES Act was passed, it was announced that the government was already taking steps to speed the development and manufacture of vaccines to prevent COVID-19. That same day, Johnson & Johnson issued a press release stating that they had received a government grant of $1 billion for vaccine development.[13] The company anticipated having a vaccine in production within a year—far quicker than the standard 5 to 10 years generally required to develop a vaccine. Dozens of other companies have been given much of the other $27 billion for drug and vaccine development. Once vaccines have

71

been developed, the government will fund the testing. The vaccines will be nearly all taxpayer funded, providing a rich bounty for the vaccine makers once the vaccines are sold and distributed.

In addition to big corporations getting free taxpayer money to develop and test their products, the officers and shareholders of these companies are reaping a fortune. After the WHO declared COVID-19 a global pandemic on March 11, 2020, stock markets collapsed around the world. While the value of most companies sank, the value of publically traded healthcare companies developing COVID-19 vaccines, drugs, and testing kits surged, creating new billionaires and boosting the fortunes of others.

The most notable new billionaire is Stéphane Bancel, the CEO of Moderna, the first company to begin human COVID-19 vaccine trials. When WHO declared a pandemic Bancel's estimated net worth was some $720 million. Since then, Moderna's stock has jumped more than 103 percent, lifting his personal fortune to an estimated $1.5 billion. Bancel joined the billionaire ranks on April 2, when Moderna's stock rose on the news that the firm was planning to begin phase two trials of its vaccine. By May 2020 the company's stock valuation soared to $29 billion even though the company had yet to sell any products.[14] It seems strange that much of the funding for Moderna's vaccine came from US taxpayers, who will end up having to pay for a vaccine that made Bancel a billionaire.

Over a period of just 7 weeks, 9 billionaires have enriched their fortunes through soaring stock prices. Those who have profited the most include French billionaire Alain Mérieux, founder of diagnostic test maker BioMérieux, and Seo Jung-Jin, CEO of South Korean biopharmaceutical firm Celltrion, who are both about $1.5 billion richer.[15] BioMérieux and DiaSorin are key players in the production of COVID-19 testing kits; both firms were selling hundreds of thousands of testing kits each week during the height of the pandemic. Some testing kits were selling online for about

$150 each, so you can imagine how much money these companies earned during the crisis.

How much money could vaccine makers pull in as a result of the coronavirus plandemic? Let's assume a vaccine proves to be successful and gets approval in the US and other major markets. If the company prices its coronavirus vaccine similarly to flu vaccines currently on the market, its list price would in the ballpark of at least $40. If we also assume at least 2 billion doses of the vaccine would be given per year, the company could be looking at annual revenue of $80 billion.[16]

GILEAD SCIENCES

During a crisis there is always the risk of price gouging of essential products. In a pandemic that could be medical supplies and drugs.

If only a couple of hundred people worldwide needed a drug, it is reasonable for the drug maker to charge a premium price to recoup the money spent in research, development, and testing. The more people who need a drug the less expensive it can be for the manufacturer to recoup his investment and make a profit. If a billion people need the drug, as might be the case with a pandemic, it should be priced accordingly like any other commonly used drug. If the drug maker used taxpayer money in the development of the drug, it should be even cheaper. Don't bet on it. Drug makers will try to get away with as much profit as they can. Gilead Sciences' antiviral drug remdesivir is a classic example.

Before remdesivir was approved, Dr. Fauci praised it highly, referring to it as the most effective treatment for COVID-19 currently available. To back up his praise he cited the success of a study conducted by the NIAID, the origination he heads. As soon as the drug was approved by the FDA, the company's value jumped by $12 billion, earning the stockholders a handsome profit.[17]

In June, 2020, Gilead Sciences, announced they would charge US hospitals $529 per dose, for a total of $3,120 for a patient with private insurance, with most patients needing 6 doses over 5 days. A lower price of $390 per dose will be offered to other governments in other countries due to agreements made between Gilead and drug manufacturers to produce remdesivir at a significantly lower cost.[18]

That same month, the US government bought more than 500,000 treatment courses of the antiviral drug, representing the manufacturer's entire production capacity for three months. At $3,120 per course that comes to more than $1.5 billion for just this initial purchase. How much of that is profit? The production costs for remdesivir are estimated to be $0.93 for one day's treatment, or less than $6 for an entire 5-day course. Patients receiving the drug end up paying for it twice; once through their taxes and again through the hospital bill.

With these prices, somebody is making a killing here. But it gets even worse. The US consumer group Public Citizen estimates taxpayers in the US, Europe, and Asia contributed $70.5 million in development costs for remdesivir.[19] Much of the research came from the US government along with generous government grants, which begs the question of whether remdesivir should be in the public domain. Instead, Gilead charges a premium price for the drug and maintains a monopoly on sales, holding patients in 70 countries, the latest of which won't expire until 2036.

In contrast, hydroxychloroquine's patent expired years ago and can be manufactured by anyone. It has proven to be effective against COVID-19 without causing any serious adverse effects, and costs about $20 for the complete treatment. Keep in mind that hydroxychloroquine has proven to save lives in clinical studies. Remdesivir, on the other hand, failed to save any lives in clinical studies. Yet, hydroxychloroquine is hotly discouraged, while remdesivir is praised and promoted as a "game changer." Why would a costly drug of questionable worth that is accompanied by serious side effects be promoted while a cheap, safe alternative is discredited? Again, follow the money. Hydroxychloroquine essentially eliminates the need for other antiviral medications or vaccines that are under development that have the potential to generate billions in revenue.

MODERNA

Although vaccines take years to develop, Moderna, Inc., had a COVID-19 vaccine ready and available for clinical testing on March 16, 2020, just 5 days after the new coronavirus was declared a global pandemic by the WHO and only 42 days after the genetic sequence of the virus was posted by Chinese scientists on an open-access website. It is curious how Moderna was able to develop a new vaccine in just 6 weeks, particularly since no one previously has been able to develop an effective vaccine for coronaviruses. Was it possible that they could have had access to critical information about the virus long before the outbreak occurred? If so, how did they get it and from whom?

Moderna, headquartered in Cambridge, Massachusetts, was founded by a group of investors in September 2010. French businessman, Stéphane Bancel, formerly the CEO of the biotech firm BioMérieux, was hired as the chief executive officer of the company in 2011. The focus of the company is drug and vaccine development with a particular interest in RNA viruses, which includes coronaviruses.

Much of their research involves inserting synthetic messenger RNA (mRNA) into living cells of patients that would reprogram the cells to create their own defense. It is a novel technique abandoned by several large pharmaceutical and biotech companies which were unable to overcome the dangerous side-effects of getting RNA into cells. As of November 2020, no mRNA drug has been approved for human use.

By 2016 Moderna had received $550 million in funding, which included $240 million from AstraZeneca, $125 million from Alexion, $100 million from Merck, and $20 million from the Bill & Melinda Gates Foundation.[20] That year they announced they would begin human testing on 6 drugs—the first of the company's products to reach this point. Four years later there has been no test results published, no products available, and no explanation. Were the tests failures? That would explain why they said nothing more.

Most companies are normally quick to publish their research and establish themselves, build a reputation in the industry, and attract investors and collaborators. Moderna, however, has a reputation for secrecy and little of its work has ever been published, and none peer-reviewed or scientifically validated, an approach that has many scientists questioning what is going on at the company.[21] Some even question if the company is even legitimate, making comparisons to Theranos, another biotech firm that collected hundreds of millions in investments based on fraudulent data.[22] The founder of the company had amassed a personal fortune of $4.5 billion before her deception was exposed.

Although Moderna holds many patents, by 2020 the company had yet to bring any products to market. Their COVID-19 vaccine is the first and only product to reach any substantial clinical trial. It seems rather suspicious that their only product to date is one that has come along at just the opportune time, beating the competition by months or years, and promises to solve the COVID-19 crisis. Even after Moderna began testing their COVID-19 vaccine, they have withheld data from the trials, which is unusual for studies like this. Are they trying to hide something from us?

Moderna isn't even the real developer of the vaccine. The vaccine was the result of a joint effort with scientists at the National Institute of Allergy and Infectious Diseases (NIAID), the organization headed by Dr. Fauci. It is apparent that Fauci was involved in the vaccine's development and may even share in the profits from it, either from royalties on patents or from the increasing value of company stocks. In April, Moderna was awarded $483 million by the US government to accelerate the development of their coronavirus vaccine, some of which may end up going Fauci's way in the form of consulting fees. It is suspiciously evident that Fauci has his fingerprints all over this pandemic; from his involvement in gain-of-function research on the coronavirus, funding of viral mutation research at the Wuhan Institute of Virology and vaccine research at Moderna, and his personal involvement in the development of the vaccine, to his insistence that we continue to isolate ourselves at home and keep certain businesses and schools closed until a vaccine is ready.

8

How Dangerous is COVID-19?

SOUNDING THE ALARM

As soon as the pandemic was declared the media was in a frenzy, blaring out dire warnings of alarm. Newspapers printed headlines such as "Death Toll Rises," "Coroner's Office Brace for Coronavirus Fatalities," and "President Declares National Emergency." You would think we were reliving the Spanish Flu pandemic or the bubonic plague that ravaged Europe in the 14th century.

Governments worldwide have responded with more aggressive and comprehensive measures to contain this virus than any pandemic in history. In the interest of public health, it's better to overreact to a crisis like this than underreact. Of course, the media have a duty to fully cover it, but the media thrive on crises, real and imagined, and have a tendency to sensationalize. Individual media outlets don't want to be upstaged by their competitors. Each tries to outdo the other with the most ostentatious news stories, creating a national crisis where one may not exist.

Elected officials, bureaucrats, and healthcare officials at all levels of government especially fear under-reacting. As the virus spreads, they'll be held accountable for precautions they didn't take that other officials did. If one school shuts down, others will follow suit. School boards and college administrators will be held accountable if a large number of their students become sick while other schools are closed. Many businesses, government offices, and places of worship have followed suit, many under government edict. Lockdown orders have been put in place in many cities and countries, restricting travel outside of the home for all except those who provide essential services.

Because of the media fearmongering and the government's hyper-reaction to save face, people were frightened and even panicked. Some to the point of hysteria hording items such as toilet paper, sanitizing wipes, and food. Store shelves were left bare. Others were forced to go without.

The world has survived more serious crises. This isn't the bubonic plague that killed half of Europe's population or the Spanish Flu that killed more than 50 million people worldwide. Yes, hundreds of thousands of people worldwide have become sick. Several thousand have died. There is reason for concern, but the situation is not nearly as dire as it has been portrayed by the media and government officials. In truth, this pandemic is no more serious than the annual flu—which never gets near as much publicity or fanfare.

DANGER OVERINFLATED

When COVID-19 first surfaced in China and began spreading to other countries there was a legitimate reason to worry. This is a new virus that has never been seen in humans and we did not know how deadly it was or how quickly it could spread. Since no one had been exposed to this particular virus before, we assumed that nobody had immunity to it. It had the potential to turn into a worldwide catastrophe. Now we can look back, we have a better understanding of its character and its potential for harm. It turns out that our initial worries were overblown. COVID-19 is a problem for sure, but not nearly as much as was believed or as much as it has been portrayed by the media.

Initial estimates for the death rate of COVID-19 ranged from 2 to 4 percent. Based on this preliminary data, newscasters and reporters made comparisons between the mortality rate of the annual flu and COVID-19. The mortality rate of the flu is often quoted as being 0.1 percent, and therefore, COVID-19 was described as being more than 20 to 40 times as deadly as the flu. However, the preliminary data used to estimate the coronavirus death rates were misleading. Death rates are accurately based on the total number of people who became infected and the number of those who died. In contrast, the death rates that were being reported were based on the number of confirmed cases from people seeking medical aid after becoming ill, not the total number of cases. The vast majority of people infected do not experience any symptoms, and therefore, have not been accounted for in calculating the true mortality rate.

According to the latest research, as many as 86 percent of those infected with COVID-19 have no symptoms.[1] That's right, the vast majority of people who have the virus aren't even aware of it. Their bodies are strong enough to fight off the virus without experiencing any discomfort or ill affect.

Considering that 86 percent show few or no symptoms, looking at confirmed cases and deaths, we find that the actual mortality rate for COVID-19 to be closer to 0.05 percent, half of that credited to the annual flu.

Let's compare the mortality rate among those people who become sick enough to be hospitalized. Keep in mind that virtually all those who were not sick enough to be admitted to the hospital eventually recovered; for them COVID-19 was just a transient illness like most other seasonal viruses. The Centers for Disease Control and Prevention (CDC) estimates that during the previous year's flu season (2018-2019), 35.5 million Americans were infected. Out of this number 16.5 million felt sick enough to seek medical attention; 490,600 people were hospitalized, and 34,200 people died. Influenza A viruses (H1N1 and H3N2) were

80

the predominate circulating viruses during the 2018-2019 flu season. The CDC classified that year's flu as moderate in severity across all age groups. In other words, the death and morbidity rate that season was typical for any given flu season.[2]

Keeping in mind that the mortality rate among hospitalized patients is far higher than that among all those who become infected, we can compare the severity of influenza A with COVID-19 by looking at the number of patients who were affected enough to be hospitalized and then died. Of the 490,000 patients that were hospitalized with influenza that season, 34,200 died, resulting in a mortality rate of 7 percent among the most severely affected patients. In comparison, of the first 138 patients hospitalized in Wuhan with COVID-19, just 6 died, indicating a mortality rate of 4.3 percent—approximately half the death rate as influenza A among hospitalized patients. Again, a fatality rate nearly half that of the flu seems to be more accurate.

Population samples from China, Italy, and the US provide further evidence. Around January 31, 2020, planes were sent to evacuate citizens from Wuhan, China. When those planes landed, the passengers were tested for COVID-19 and quarantined. After 14 days, the percentage who tested positive was 0.9 percent. If this was the prevalence in the greater Wuhan area on January 31, then, with a population of about 20 million, greater Wuhan had 178,000 infections, about 30 times more than the number of reported cases. The fatality rate, then, would be at least 10 times lower than estimates based on reported cases.

Vò is a town in the province of Padua, Italy. On March 6, 2020, all 3,300 residents of Vò were tested for COVID-19. Ninety tested positive for the virus, indicating a prevalence of 2.7 percent. It can be reasonably assumed that the entire province of Padua would have a similar percentage of infected people. Padua had 198 reported cases. Applying that prevalence rate of 2.7 percent to the entire population of Padua (955,000), that would mean 26,000 people were actually infected with the virus, more than 130 times the number reported. This illustrates that far more people are infected than those who reported feeling sick, which is in agreement with the 86 percent of positive case experiencing no symptoms. Although Italy has reported a fatality rate of 8 percent based on confirmed cases, according the above figures, the actual mortality rate in closer to 0.06 percent.

The COVID-19 outbreak in Wuhan China was first made public on December 31, 2019. By that time, however, the virus had already infected hundreds and perhaps even thousands of people in Wuhan and many other cities in China. The first known case in the US occurred in Washington state on January 15 by a man who had returned from visiting relatives in Wuhan. It is likely that the coronavirus had entered the US even before that time as many other travelers had returned to the US from China before the outbreak was made public. COVID-19 has proven to be highly contagious and it is believed that the number of infected people doubles about every 3 days. If the first infected traveler came to the US on January 1, by March 9, the virus could have passed to as many as 6 million Americans. According to the CDC, as of March 23, there were 499 COVID-19 related deaths in the US. If 6 million people were infected, the mortality rate would be 0.01 percent. Today, the infection rate would be far higher, yet death rates have been no worse than the seasonal flu.

According to the CDC, as of March 31, 2020 there had been 180,271 reported cases of COVID-19 in the US and 3,573 deaths. In contrast, over the same period of time there were 38 to 54 million cases of the flu, resulting in 24,000 to 62,000 deaths.[3] COVID-19 doesn't even compare to the flu in terms of number of cases or deaths caused. The CDC stopped recording flu statistics on their website after the first week in April. Since April, the number of deaths attributed to COVID-19 has been greatly inflated and includes most flu cases, making any further comparison unreliable.

Since April testing isn't even necessary to be classified as a COVID case. All you need is a simple upper respiratory infection and you will likely be classified as a COVID-19 case, which artificially inflates the totals.

At the beginning of the pandemic hospitals began gearing up for an onslaught of COVID-19 cases. All medical procedures and surgeries were canceled to free up the medical staff and beds to handle the expected wave of pandemic victims. The doctors and staff waited and waited. A few patients experiencing respiratory complaints were admitted, assumedly because they had COVID-19, but there was no flood of coronavirus patients. The expected flood turned into a meandering stream.

At first, "The clarion call was to clear the hospitals of patients," says UK physician and bestselling author Malcolm Kendrick. But the hospitals were never filled. In fact, they were mostly empty with the medical staff sitting around idle. "There was a point when my local hospital was a quarter full. Staff were wandering around with nothing to do. You hear this idea that all NHS staff have been working 20 times as hard as they have ever done. This is complete nonsense. An awful lot of people have been standing around wondering what the hell to do with themselves. A&E (the emergency room) has never been so quiet." This situation is true for most all hospitals.[4]

DOES NOT KILL INDISCRIMINATELY

Although potentially deadly, COVID-19 does not kill indiscriminately, it carefully chooses its victims. Like a sniper, it targets a select group of individuals—those with compromised immune systems. Young, healthy people are less affected; they may acquire the virus but their bodies are capable of fighting it off with little or no symptoms, leaving them with a lifelong immunity to the virus.

As is the case with most seasonal viral infections, the elderly are always the most vulnerable because they are the ones who have the lowest resistance to infectious disease. They are the ones who need to take the greatest precautions. Although younger people may become ill, they almost always recover. Our bodies are conditioned to fight off infection. We do it all the time, even when we are not aware of it. It is a constant battle with the microbes with which we share our environment.

The most vulnerable are those who have underlying health problems that lower their resistance to infections. Although anyone with low immunity, regardless of their age, may be susceptible, age is a major factor. With advancing age, resistance to disease declines and health conditions, such as diabetes, emphysema, and chronic bronchitis, become more common. Any chronic disease will tax the immune system making a person more vulnerable to infection.

Although COVID-19 struck fear into the hearts of people of all ages, it was the elderly who were at greatest risk; the risk declines dramatically with age. During the first few months of the pandemic very few children and adolescents under the age of 19 became ill (less than 0.2 percent) with no reported deaths in the US.

According to the CDC, during the first few months of the COVID-19 pandemic people in the US who were 65 years of age or older accounted for 31 percent of the cases reported, 45 percent of the hospitalizations, 53 percent of the intensive care unit (ICU) admissions, and 80 percent of the deaths. Those people who were 85 or older experienced the highest percentage of severe outcomes. Although older people accounted for only 31 percent of those who reported being sick, they made up 80 percent of the deaths.[5]

The death rate in a given country depends a lot on the age-structure, who are the people infected, and how they are managed. For people younger than 45, the infection fatality rate is almost 0 percent. For 45 to 70, it is about 0.05 to 0.3 percent. For those above 70, it escalates to 1 percent.[6] The fatality rate is highest in persons aged 85 and older, ranging from 10 to 27 percent. The risk is greatest among frail, debilitated elderly people with multiple health problems, especially if they reside in long-term healthcare facilities. The number of people in nursing homes accounts for less than 1 percent of the US population, but a staggering 43.4 percent of all COVID-19 deaths.

Among the general population, COVID-19 has proven to be no more serious than a case of the flu. In children 15 years of age and under, the risk is nearly zero. The chance of dying from a lightning strike is one in 700,000. The chance of dying of COVID-19 in that age group in 1 in 3.5 million.[7] The most vulnerable are the elderly and those with preexisting health conditions.

According to Dr. Steven Shapiro, chief medical and scientific officer of the University of Pittsburgh Medical Center: "Our outcomes are similar to the state of Pennsylvania, where the median age of death from COVID-19 is 84 years old. The few younger patients who died all had significant preexisting conditions. Very few children were infected and none died. Minorities in our communities fared equally well as others, but we know that this is not the case nationally. In sum, this is a disease of the elderly, sick, and poor."[8] It is not a disease of young or relatively healthy individuals.

YOU MAY ALREADY BE IMMUNE

From the very start of the COVID-19 pandemic there has been a great deal of stress placed on developing a vaccine. A vaccination is promoted as the only solution to this pandemic.

As the scientific community frantically searches for a new vaccine to fight COVID-19, the need for a vaccine may not be so critical. Researchers have recently discovered that previous exposure to some forms of the common cold can provide long-term immunity against COVID-19. Studies have shown that some 60 to 80 percent of the population may already be immune to the coronavirus.[9=80]

Every fall as cold and flu season rolls around millions

of people experience the sinus congestion, coughing and sneezing, and general lack of energy associated with the common cold. The common cold is caused by a virus—a number of viruses actually. There are some 200 viruses that can cause colds. Among these, human rhinoviruses (HRVs) are the most common, accounting for more than half of the cold-like illnesses that occur annually. The next most common are coronaviruses, responsible for as many as 30 percent of cases. The rest are caused by various other respiratory viruses.

Coronaviruses that are associated with the common cold cause only a mild upper respiratory tract infection typical of a common cold and are resolved on their own after a week or two. Like rhinoviruses and influenza, they appear seasonally each year and are found worldwide.

SARS-CoV-2, which causes COVID-19, has similar genetic features as other coronaviruses, including the human coronaviruses that are known to cause the common cold. If an individual has been previously exposed to any of the coronaviruses, the body develops memory T cells, which become a defense system when other coronaviruses attack the body, resulting in immunity against the viruses.

T cells, a type of white blood cell, is a prominent part of the immune system, priming the body to quickly respond to invasion from viruses and other organisms. Because of their ability to create lasting defense against viruses, they are called memory cells.

Medical researchers worldwide are actively seeking to develop antivirals and vaccines to fight COVID-19. As a result of this research, a number of studies have discovered that people who have been exposed to other coronaviruses, such as SARS and human coronaviruses, specifically HCoV-OC43 and HCoV-HKU1, have antibodies that protect them against COVID-19.[11] According to a team of researchers from Duke University and the National University of Singapore, immune protection against COVID-19 derived from a previous coronavirus infection can last at least 17 years and perhaps for life.[12] In contrast, the vaccines that are currently being developed for COVID-19 produce such low levels of antibodies that multiple injections are required and the immunity that is achieved wears off in time so that revaccination would likely be needed every year.

At the onset of the COVID-19 pandemic it was predicted that tens of millions of people would be infected. However, the actual number of cases has been far lower than anticipated. Since human coronaviruses are among the seasonal infections that come and go every year, many people have been infected and have developed a natural long-lasting immunity. This may have been why the number of people infected with COVID-19 has been lower than expected.[13]

That cold you had last year or the year before, may have been the thing that kept you healthy and unaffected by COVID-19 this year. Although many government and public health officials are insisting we need a vaccine before we can get back to normal, most of us already have immunity to the coronavirus.

Hundreds of thousands of people have tested positive for COVID-19. While it has been found that many of the testing kits used were flawed and gave false positives in many cases, another problem is that if you tested positive it may have been because you had a cold and not COVID-19. Millions of people worldwide come down with the cold every year. Everybody has been so frightened that if they suspect any signs of a possible respiratory infection they immediately suspect COVID-19. When they get an antibody test and receive a positive result they think they have the coronavirus and they are added to the growing number of cases of COVID-19 that are used to scare us. In many, and maybe even most cases, you may have a coronavirus infection, not SARS-CoV-2, but one of the more benign human coronavirus that contribute to the common cold each year.

An infection by one of the human coronavirus produce

antibodies similar to those of COVID-19. If you test positive to COVID-19 it could mean you simply have a cold. Even the CDC acknowledges this fact stating, "...a positive result means that you have antibodies from an infection with a virus from the same family of viruses (called coronaviruses), such as the one that causes the common cold."[14]

Of the many millions of people worldwide testing positive to COVID-19, how many actually have COVID-19? Probably a lot fewer than we think.

9

A Misinformation Campaign

**WE ARE VICTIMS OF A MASSIVE
MISINFORMATION CAMPAIGN**

Why are lockdowns, masks, and social distancing so heavily promoted and even mandated? The reason is due to fear that people who are infected with COVID-19 but unaware of it, may be the primary spreaders of the disease.

Studies have indicated that as many as 86 percent of people who test positive for COVID-19 are asymptomatic, meaning they show no symptoms of the disease.[1] These people may act as carriers and spread the disease to others. Since there is no way, without testing, to tell if a healthy person is infected, everyone is suspect. For this reason, lockdowns, masks, and social distancing have been justified, to reduce the risk of passing the infection to others.

During a press briefing on June 8, 2020, Dr. Maria Van Kerkhove, the World Health Organization's technical lead for the COVID-19 pandemic, stated that the data they have clearly shows that asymptomatic people do not spread the virus and if it happens it is "very rare."[2]

Here is her exact statement: "From the data we have, it still seems to be rare that an asymptomatic person actually transmits onward to a secondary individual. We have a number of reports from countries who are doing very detailed contact tracing. They're following asymptomatic cases, they're following contacts and they're not finding secondary transmission onward. It is very rare—and much of that is not published in the literature. We are constantly looking at this data and we're trying to get more information from countries to truly answer this question. It still appears to be rare that an asymptomatic individual actually transmits onward."

This announcement hit like a bombshell. If asymptomatic people don't spread the virus, why is there so much emphases on wearing face masks, closing down businesses and public gatherings, self quarantining at home, and practicing social distancing? We were doing all those things in the belief that anyone could be a carrier and could pass the virus to others. Now, according to Dr. Van Kerkhove, the results of "very detailed studies" from a number of countries show that assumption to be false.

The only people who justifiably need to take measures to prevent passing the virus are those who are noticeably sick, rather than those who are feeling well. Eliminating these restrictions and allowing people to go back to work, open up restaurants and stores to full capacity, and attend church, sporting events, and other gatherings would be the sensible thing to do. Doing so, would erase nearly all the fear and panic from the virus that the mainstream and social media have tried so hard to create. Life would go back to normal and the pandemic would become a fading memory. If this happened it would destroy the widespread feelings of fear and hopelessness that Bill Gates and Big Pharma have tried so hard to create, which could greatly hinder the acceptance and compulsion for the mass vaccination campaign they have been building.

When Van Kerkhove made these statements, she was simply answering a question put to her at the press conference. She was answering the question truthfully according to her knowledge. Apparently, the directors of the WHO and their funders, namely Bill Gates and Big Pharma, were outraged to see one of their scientists publically admit that all the safety measures that they had been so adamantly pushing, were useless. Van Kerkhove was undoubtedly reprimanded and instructed to backtrack and "clarify" her statement.

Within 24 hours Van Kerkhove publicly announced that her comments on the previous day were not clearly stated and were misunderstood. What she meant to say was that only a few small studies showed low transmission rates from asymptomatic people. She said she failed to mention the computer modeling programs, which are based on assumptions, that estimated a wide range of transmission, some of which estimated that asymptomatic transmission up to 40 percent. In other words, what she was saying was that independent research by several countries doing detailed tracking transmission studies, collecting real data not estimates, should be ignored and, instead, we should believe the estimates produced by computer models that are based on nothing more than assumptions. The entire rational for social distancing, wearing of face masks, and shutting down businesses is based on inaccurate estimates from computer models, not real data. The actual data says the opposite. We have all been lied to.

It is interesting to note that all of the misleading computer modeling projections for the COVID-19 pandemic have come out of the Imperial College in Great Britain and the Institute for Health Metrics and Evaluation located in Gates' hometown in Seattle. Both institutions receive funding from WHO, which in turn, is heavily funded by the Bill & Melinda Gates Foundation.[3] In fact, the Institute for Health Metrics and Evaluation was launched in 2007 by a $105 million grant from the Gates Foundation.

I highly recommend that you watch this video https://www.youtube.com/watch?v=EnpCOOmUtBs before it is deleted from Youtube. It shows Van Kerkhove's original comments and her disjointed attempt on the following day to rationalize her statements and conform to the WHO's misinformation campaign.

We are told to stay a certain distance apart to avoid passing the virus to others. In the US it is 6 feet. Why 6 feet? There is no strong evidence that 6 feet is better than 3 or even 1 foot. The distance varies from country to county. For example, in the UK, Spain, and Italy it is 2 meters (6.5 feet); in Germany, Poland, and Netherlands it is 1.5 meters (5 feet); and in Austria, Norway, and Sweden it is 1 meter (3.25 feet). After reviewing a WHO paper on social distancing, two Oxford professors, Carl Heneghan and Tom Jefferson, argue that there is little proof to support the restriction. The pair, who work at Oxford University's Centre for Evidence-Based Medicine, reviewed 38 studies that focus on the effect of social distancing and stated that "much of the evidence informing policy in the outbreak is poor quality." Only 1 study looked specifically at coronavirus infections and found that distancing of 2 meters had no effect. The same conclusion was independently arrived at by Dr. Mike Lonergan, a senior statistician and epidemiologist at the University of Dundee.[4]

There is additional evidence that asymptomatic people do not spread the virus and that social distancing and masks are unnecessary. Despite nationwide adherence to social distancing and lockdowns, these measures have proven to have been a dismal failure. The vast majority of those people who come down with the virus are those who have strictly followed these guidelines, not the ones who have been out and about mingling with others.

New York Governor Andrew Cuomo says that it is "shocking" to discover that 66 percent of new hospitalizations appear to have been among people "largely sheltering at home."

"We thought maybe they were taking public transportation," he said, "but actually no, because these people were literally at home."[5]

"Much of this comes down to what you do to protect yourself," he continues. "Everything closed down, government has done everything it could, society has done everything it could."

It's your fault, he says to the hospitalized New Yorkers who loyally complied with his government directive. But here is an interesting alternative theory as to why, mostly, old people who are staying at home are being hospitalized. What if the government directive to close everything down and mandate "social distancing" actually made the problem worse?

FRESH AIR AND SUNSHINE
The Spanish flu of 1918 was the most devastating viral pandemic in history, far deadlier than the coronavirus, killing between 50 million and 100 million people worldwide. Research at the time demonstrated that patients who were exposed to fresh air and sunshine in "open-air hospitals" had a better chance at survival.[6] The open-air hospital concept was used in sanatoriums that were popular during the late 1800s and early 1900s. At these hospitals patients were exposed to ample sunlight and fresh air as part of their treatment. These hospitals treated patients with influenza, pneumonia, tuberculosis and other diseases. In those days, tuberculosis—a potentially deadly bacterial respiratory infection—was a major cause of death. Open-air hospitals were the most effective treatment of the day, reducing mortality rates by half in comparison to patients receiving orthodox treatment.[7]

The Spanish flu pandemic began while World War I was still raging. Many soldiers and sailors were affected. Military hospitals treated infected soldiers and sailors by the thousands, many of which were housed in tents, which were essentially open-air hospitals. At Camp Brooks open-air hospital near Boston, medical officer Major Thomas F. Harrington studied the history of his patients and found that the worst cases came from those who worked in the parts of ships that were most badly ventilated.[8] Thus, suggesting being in a closed environment with limited access to fresh air and sunshine contributed to the onset of the disease.

The curative effects of fresh air were investigated at length by the British physiologist Sir Leonard Hill in the years following World War I. He reported favorably on the effects of the sun and air when judiciously applied, particularly for tuberculosis. In 1919, Hill wrote in the *British Medical Journal* that the best way to combat influenza infection was deep breathing of cool air and sleeping, under warm covers, in the open where fresh air was available.[9] Fresh air, sunshine, and the warmth of the sun were considered the keys to the success of these hospitals.

The surgeon general of the Massachusetts State Guard, William A. Brooks, had no doubt that open-air methods were effective at the Brooks hospital, despite opposition from those who expressed little faith in the therapy. Skeptics felt that patients would get the same benefits if the windows of a conventional ward were open or the patients were put in a hospital "sun parlor." Brooks, however, held that patients did not do as well in an ordinary hospital, no matter how well the rooms were ventilated or how much time they spent in the sun parlor, as they did outdoors. He reported that in one general hospital with 76 cases, 20 patients died within three days and 17 nurses fell ill. By contrast, the regimen adopted at the camp reduced the fatality of hospital cases from 40 percent to about 13 percent.[10] Brooks wrote that "The efficacy of open air treatment has been absolutely proven, and one has only to try it to discover its value."[11]

Fever is one of the symptoms characteristic of COVID-19. The reason the body produces a fever is to generate heat. Most infectious microorganisms, including SARS-Cov-2, cannot tolerate too much heat. Temperatures equivalent to a low-grade fever kill the virus. During the summer months ordinary temperatures often experienced at this time would kill the virus.

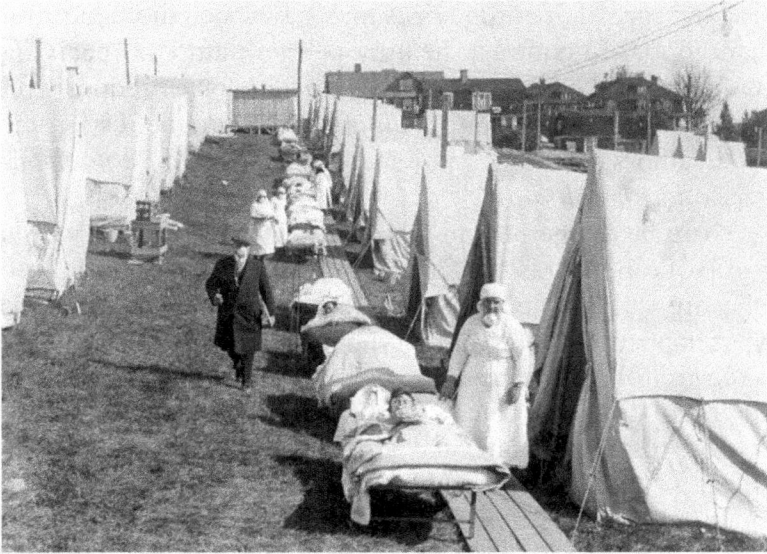

Influenza patients getting sunlight at the Camp Brooks emergency open-air hospital in Boston. Doctors found that severely ill flu patients nursed outdoors recovered better than those treated indoors.

The coronavirus does not like heat or the sun. In fact, direct sunlight kills the virus. It is well-known that sunlight is an effective disinfectant—a natural sanitizer.[12] Researchers have found that sunlight can kill SARS-Cov-2 within 34 minutes. The scientists say that when the virus has been coughed or sneezed onto surfaces, that sunlight during the summer is extremely effective in killing it. Without sun exposure the virus can live on surfaces for up to a day.[13]

Sunlight is our primary source of immune boosting vitamin D. Daily exposure to the sun can provide substantial protection against COVID-19. If adequate sunlight is not available, dietary supplements can also raise vitamin D levels.

Studies on vitamin D and past success against respiratory infection at open-air hospitals strongly suggests that the mandatory stay-at-home orders issued in hopes of stopping the spread of coronavirus may have been more harmful than good. "In contrast, healthy people outdoors receiving sunlight could have been exposed to a lower viral dose with more chances for mounting an efficient immune response," state authors of a study published in the journal *Photochemistry and Photobiology.*[14]

You have one person who is infected locked up with a group of others, it is only a matter of time before all of those who are vulnerable will become infected as well. This is what happened in the nursing homes. Infected people were taken to nursing homes where they spread the infection to others. In other healthcare facilities the virus was carried in by new residents, staff, and visiting family and friends. In all cases, the virus spread like wildfire. However, just being in a nursing home does not make you susceptible to infection. You must also have an underlying health problem that lowers your ability to fight off the infection. While healthcare facilities were the most heavily hit by the virus, most of the residents did not become sick. Even elderly people, who are in relatively good health for their age, can be immune to the virus.

Mandating that people say at home, locking down businesses, closing parks and beaches, and preventing people, including residents of nursing homes, from doing any outdoor activities where they can benefit from the fresh air and sunshine has actually increased the risk and severity of COVID-19. That is why the majority of those who have been sickened with COVID-19 are the ones who have isolated themselves as instructed. If you wanted to get as many people as possible sick during an outbreak, sheltering in place is one of the best ways to accomplish it. Enacting laws to enforce it with the threat of fines or jail time, as was often done, would make sure the population complied and a maximum number of people infected. Dr. Anthony Fauci and other public health officials who advocated self-isolation should have known what would happen. Perhaps they did.

The incident with the USS Theodore Roosevelt demonstrates what the virus does in a closed environment among relatively healthy people. The virus broke out after the ship left port and was at sea. The crew lived in close quarters with each other, so there was no social distancing, masks, or massive quarantining. Out of a total of 4,800 crewmembers, 1,102 became infected. However only 7 required hospitalization, with 1 death. Such a low transmission rate contrasts greatly with the computer models that have predicted high transmissibility and fatality.

The actual infection rate was 23 percent, and among those infected, the fatality rate was 0.09 percent. Among the Roosevelt's entire crew of assumedly healthy and able-bodied sailors, on a floating Petri dish, during the thick of a viral outbreak, which on the mainland had shut down all schools and placed healthy citizens across America under house-arrest, the fatality rate was a mere 0.002 percent. In view of these facts, it seems more than obvious that there is little sense in social distancing.

DEATH RATES MISLEADING

If you look at the statistics the number of people who have died from COVID-19 seems astronomical. As of July 2020, more than 130,000 deaths have been attributed to COVID-19 in the US.[15] While this number of deaths appears frightening, in reality it is not that significant. In comparison, 647,000 Americans die each year from heart disease, 606,520 die from cancer, 140,00 die from stroke, another 140,000 die from chronic obstructive pulmonary disease (COPD), and 38,000 die from automobile accidents.

Death from these other causes have been fairly consistent over the past few years. Therefore, in 2020 you would expect the additional deaths from COVID-19 to greatly increase the total death count—at least by 130,000. However that is not the case. The total all-cause mortality is not significantly different than in previous years. The reason why total deaths are not higher in 2020 is because the COVID-19 death statistics have been artificially inflated. Numerous deaths caused by heart disease, cancer, stroke, influenza, and even accidents and suicide have been reported as CO-VID-19 related. People who already had terminal illnesses who displayed any signs of respiratory illness, such as a cough or fever, were assumed to have COVID-19 and when they died, that was put on their death certificates. Therefore, many thousands of deaths from other causes, that would have occurred whether they had COVID-19 or not, were attributed to COVID-19.

The additional deaths caused by COVID-19 should have caused a marked upward spike in the overall death rate. But the death rate has actually gone down in comparison to previous years. According to the American Institute of Economic Research "The latest figures on overall death rates from all causes show no increase at all. Deaths are lower than in 2019, 2018, 2017 and 2015, slightly higher than in 2016. Any upward bias is imparted by population growth...all deaths are down, it must mean people are being recorded as dying from other things at smaller rates than usual. Deaths from other causes are simply being ascribed to the coronavirus."[16]

Dr. Fauci and co-conspirators are insisting that before children can return to school, restaurants and churches can be filled to capacity, and everything go back to normal, that a vaccine be developed and everyone be vaccinated. Social distancing is crucial to the master plan to force vaccination on us all. Social distancing, which includes wearing masks, limiting the number of people allowed in businesses and parks, and isolating ourselves at home, has been instigated to cause us great discomfort, anger, and fear. This is done purposely so that when a vaccine comes available the majority of us will demand that everyone be vaccinated in order for the restrictions to be lifted. Those who question the safety of the vaccines or hesitate to be vaccinated, will be publically shammed, severely criticized as selfish and ignorant, and possibly even physically abused until they submit to the pressure. Many parents who have questioned vaccinations for their children in the past have already experienced this type of thing. Because of all of the trauma caused by the senseless distancing mandates, persecution will be intensified.

The media and public health officials will continue to promote the scenario that coronavirus is a highly contagious and deadly infection and that the only thing that will save us is a vaccine. The media will continue to blare out troubling headlines citing new deaths, rising infection rates, and the dangers of not obeying social distancing. Their goal is to keep you scared and willing to submit to and even demand mass vaccinations.

10

Plandemic Master Plan

The steps taken to address the COVID-19 pandemic were never about public safety or public concern, but rather about power and greed. Those who profited the most were the rich stockholders and directors of major pharmaceutical and biotech companies and their patsies in positions of authority over us who dished out all of the misinformation and recommended the draconian regulations. The way to find the source to a problem is to follow the money and the money clearly leads to these billionaires. They claim any link between them and the pandemic is a senseless conspiracy theory and anyone, including scientists, who question the measures taken are quacks. Is it a conspiracy that these billionaires racked in hundreds of millions of dollars, in some cases billions of dollars, when the rest of the world was reeling in the worst recession since the Great Depression and millions of people were thrown out of work? The fact is, these people who control our healthcare have enriched themselves at our expense.

To make matters worse, we could see a repeat of all this in coming years. We are told that SARS-Cov-2 is mutating, suggesting that it can transform into another strain of coronavirus that may cause a new pandemic next year or the year after. Whether SARS-CoV-2 mutates naturally or another mutated form of the virus is "accidentally" released from Wuhan Institute of Virology or another lab, we may see a repeat of what has happened in the near future. The people behind the pandemic will reap another fortune.

This pandemic didn't come about by chance. It was a carefully orchestrated event that had been in the making for years, perhaps as far back as 2010 or 2011 as evidenced by the founding of Moderna. The master plan for the plandemic required several steps and many players. The face of the pandemic, Anthony Fauci, was not likely one of the instigators, but he was surly a willing participant and key figure. He was merely a puppet with others pulling the strings.

Below is a summary of the major steps that were taken to pull off the biggest health scam in history.

Financial Backers

Gather together a group of billionaires from around the world who have financial interests in the pharmaceutical and biomedical industries and work out the details of the plandemic.

Find A Novel Virus

Central to the plan is the creation of a virus that is highly contagious and potentially lethal. The virus must be different enough from previous pathogens so that everyone is vulnerable and no medicines or vaccines are available to fight it. Gain-of-function research was already in the works to provide a suitable pathogen.

Control the Media

Gain influence over the editorial content of the major medical journals and media outlets, including social media, through extensive advertising.

Control Health Organizations

With the use of donations and funding, buy the loyalty of the leaders and administrators of the world's major health organizations, including the World Health Organization (WHO), Centers for Disease Control and Prevention (CDC), National Institute of Allergy and Infectious Diseases (NIAIV), European Centre for Disease Prevention and Control (ECDC), and others. Wherever possible, install puppets in leadership positions that can be easily controlled (i.e., Tedros Adhanom Ghebreyesus, the Director General of WHO).

Use Organizations as the Mouthpiece

Using the authority and reputations of major health organizations, have them lead the charge on the pandemic, disseminating information (or misinformation) and setting policies to address the crisis. Push for wide scale vaccinations. In this way, the real instigators can hide in the background.

Control Government Authorities

Influence government civic and health authorities by promises of political contributions and donations to support the misinformation spread by the WHO and other health organizations.

Release the Virus in A County that Will Maximize its Spread

Release the virus in a country that has a great deal of international travel, a reputation for censorship, and would face international embarrassment as the point of origin. The country would take measures to hide the incident and delay any action, allowing the virus to spread beyond its borders leading to an international health crisis. China was the obvious choice as it was the source of the first SARS outbreak in 2002.

A Naturally Evolved Virus

Promote the cause of the outbreak as a naturally occurring novel virus to hide any involvement with existing laboratories and individuals. Compare its assumed origins to that of the earlier SARS virus.

Declare A Global Pandemic

Sound the alarm by declaring a global pandemic, creating fear and apprehension worldwide.

Exaggerate the Danger of the Pandemic

Use computer models based on the worse possible case scenario to estimate the number of people who could possibly become infected and die. Base all health policies and actions on these estimates. Ignore or discredit any solid facts that may contradict the computer model estimates.

Media Blitz

Funnel carefully crafted news releases and shocking statistics to the media to project the impression that everyone is in dire danger. Continue to feed the media outrageous stories and half truths to maintain universal anxiety and fear.

Censorship

Censor all natural health websites, blogs, and voices that may offer quick solutions or question the propaganda dissimilated by the media and health authorities. Encourage mainstream and social media to ignore or suppress any opposing viewpoints or data, including those from scientists and published studies. Have them rely on the WHO as the ultimate authority.

Discredit All Existing Solutions

Dissuade the use of any inexpensive product or therapy that may offer hope in the fight against the virus. Claim they are ineffective and dangerous. Publish fraudulent studies if necessary as proof.

Declare Vaccines as the Only Solution

Encourage the use of new antivirals as a means to treat an existing infection, but insist on vaccination as the only long-term solution for the prevention of the disease. Only a vaccine will stop the virus. Have normal safety studies suspended during the crisis to fast-track and cut the costs for the development of vaccines. Get hefty government grants to help fund the research.

Enact Lockdowns and Social Distancing

Have government authorities mandate harsh social distancing measures to create anxiety, fear, and anger. Arrest or fine those who disobey. Maintain the lockdowns as long as possible. Make people so frightened, miserable, angry, and financially distressed that they will gladly be vaccinated to end the madness, be willing to accept mandatory vaccination without complaint, and even compel those who hesitate to be vaccinated by intimidation and shaming.

Keep People Indoors

Compel everyone to stay at home. Close parks, beaches, and all outdoor activities to encourage compliance. Being confined to the home will keep people out of the sun, so they cannot produce vitamin D, away from fresh air, and reduce physical activity all of which depress immune function and makes them more susceptible to the virus, thus increasing the number of cases and inflating the statistics.

Inflate the Numbers

Increase the number of cases and deaths by including those who have the flu or other respiratory illnesses into the COVID-19 count. Have testing labs and kits give positive results to the virus whether the patient has the virus or not.

Silence the Skeptics

When people bring up the failings, errors, and inconsistencies of the advice given by the WHO, and mention involvement with Big Pharma and others, brush them aside as conspiracy theorists. Anyone who doesn't agree with the information fed to us by Dr. Fauci and the WHO are dismissed as fanatics, idiots, and wackos, believing in some type of global conspiracy. Sidestep questions and doubts by calling those who voice concerns conspiracy theorists and quacks that everybody should ignore. Even when some of these people are respected scientists.

Enjoy Instant Wealth and Repeat
The final step in the Plandemic Master Plan is to cash in on the financial windfall and sit back and enjoy. Repeat with another virus at a future date.

With all the paranoid emphasis on social distancing, wearing of masks, and sanitizing everything to prevent deaths, why has it not wiped out the homeless who don't bathe or sanitize their hands or wash their clothes, don't social distance, don't wear masks, live in unsanitary environments, and are generally undernourished and most vulnerable to infection?

In 2019, 1.5 million people worldwide died of tuberculosis. Tuberculoses is highly contagious and passes in the same manner as COVID-19. Why were you not wearing a mask during the tuberculoses pandemic? You were endangering health and public safety along with billions of other people around the globe. So why didn't you wear a mask? I'll tell you why. Because the media didn't tell you to wear a mask. There was no tuberculosis pandemic, any more than there was a coronavirus pandemic.

As of September 2020 over 180,000 deaths have been atributed to COVID-19 in the US. If the virus has killed more than 180,000 people, why are the total overall deaths for 2020 lower in 4 out of the previous 5 years? How can there be so many COVID-19 deaths, yet total number of deaths be so low? Obviously, deaths that normally occur from other causes have been credited to COVID-19.

If the virus is so deadly, why have the number of cases and deaths been artificially inflated? Why is there a need to lie to the public unless there was an ulterior motive behind the pandemic?

If there is a real pandemic, does it require faulty virus models, rigged test results, 80 percent false positives, inaccurate news reports, staged hospital overruns, and manipulated death certificates? A real pandemic would not need fake news to alert us and warn us of the danger. The facts would speak for themselves.

When the government shuts down millions of small businesses but does not lay off any government employees, it is not about health. When dentists, chiropractors, and psychologists, and other health professionals are banned from practicing, but abortion clinics are deemed essential, it is not about your health. When medical treatments, such as cancer screening, chemotherapy, and hip replacement and prostate surgeries are deemed unnecessary, while hospitals operate at half capacity due to the lack of COVID-19 cases, it is not about your health. When you are forced to isolate yourself in your home, away from sunshine and fresh air and prevented from even going to parks and beaches, yet you are allowed to go out and purchase alcohol and marijuana, it is not about your health. Folks, we've been lied to on a grand scale.

The entire pandemic was a epic hoax. We were the victims. Many people who could have been helped by hydroxychloroquine, vitamin D, and other currently available treatments were denied access to or discouraged from using these treatments, resulting in many needless deaths. It makes me angry and should you too, that we have been manipulated and lied to, that businesses were closed, and millions put out of work, all for the sake of enriching a bunch of billionaires and their lackeys. Many people who have blindly trusted government and health officials and the media, have been unaware of these facts.

The purpose of this book is to open people's eyes to the truth. Please consider sharing it with others so that we are not led down this disastrous route again when the next so-called pandemic hits.

Appendix

Additional Information
About COVID-19

Plandemic: An Expert Virologist Speaks Out
A video banned by YouTube now available here.
https://www.brighteon.com/91f524b4-656f-4c46-bab5-
01dea4ac1cf1

COVID Vaccine's New Lowes
This video was banned by YouTube but is available here.
https://thehighwire.com/watch/

Coronavirus May be Weakening and Could Die Out On Its Own.
https://www.dailymail.co.uk/news/article-8444151/amp/
Coronavirus-withered-aggressive-tiger-wild-cat-Italian-
scientist-claims.html?__twitter_impression=true

The CDC Confirms Remarkably Low Coronavirus Death Rate. Where is the Media?
https://www.theblaze.com/op-ed/horowitz-the-cdc-confirms-
remarkably-low-coronavirus-death-rate-where-is-the-media

Why Does COVID-19 Disproportionately Affect Older People?
https://www.aging-us.com/article/103344/text

Pandemic Reporting: is the Media Getting it Wrong?
https://www.organicconsumers.org/blog/pandemic-
reporting-media-getting-it-wrong

**AstraZeneca Starts Manufacturing COVID-19 Vaccine
Before Clinical Tests are Done: Strikes Deal with Bill
Gates-Backed Health Organizations**
https://www.marketwatch.com/amp/story/guid/B390F8B8-
A70D-11EA-9237-EF7B9133097E?cx_testId=3&cx_
testVariant=cx_2&cx_artPos=6&__twitter_impression=true

Death Statistics for COVID-19 are Insanely Wrong!
https://www.medpagetoday.com/infectiousdisease/
covid19/86967?xid=nl_mpt_DHE_2020-06-
10&eun=g1301936d0r&utm_source=Sailthru&utm_
medium=email&utm_campaign=Daily%20Headlines%20
Top%20Cat%20HeC%20%202020-06-10&utm_term=NL_
Daily_DHE_dual-gmail-definitio

YouTube Bans Mercola Videos
https://articles.mercola.com/sites/articles/
archive/2020/06/17/banned-youtube-mercola-videos.
aspx?cid_source=dnl&cid_medium=email&cid_content=a
rt1ReadMore&cid=20200617Z1&et_cid=DM567253&et_
rid=896079971

**Gates Adviser Quits Over COVID-19
Immunity Passports**
https://biohackinfo.com/news-elizabeth-renieris-id2020-
coronavirus-bill-gates-digital-certificate/?fbclid=IwAR0
4Cer6ybh6fkUn3A08nKzuccYtAeCBYgSPwGUxaAbj-
OfGAU7Cw0n3kFg

**Mandatory COVID-19 Vaccination for Adults and
Children**
https://www.nejm.org/doi/full/10.1056/
NEJMp2020926?query=TOC

Coronavirus Expert Says Americans Will be Wearing Masks for 'Several years'
https://www.foxnewsYcom/us/coronavirus-expert-says-americans-will-be-wearing-masks-for-several-years

81 Percent In COVID-19 Vaccine Trial Suffer Adverse Reactions
https://thevaccinereaction.org/2020/07/81-percent-of-clinical-trial-volunteers-suffer-reactions-to-cansino-biologics-covid-19-vaccine-that-uses-hek293-human-fetal-cell-lines/

COVID-19 Had a Lab Origin
https://www.independentsciencenews.org/health/the-case-is-building-that-covid-19-had-a-lab-origin/

Masked Science: Do Masks Protect You From COVID-19?
https://articles.mercola.com/sites/articles/archive/2020/07/15/do-masks-protect-you-from-covid-19.aspx?cid_source=dnl&cid_medium=email&cid_content=art2ReadMore&cid=20200715Z1

How a False Hydroxychloroquine Narrative Was Created
https://articles.mercola.com/sites/articles/archive/2020/07/15/hydroxychloroquine-for-coronavirus.aspx?cid_source=dnl&cid_medium=email&cid_content=art1ReadMore&cid=20200715Z1

'Trust Stamp' Vaccine Record and Payment System Rolling Out in Africa
https://www.mintpressnews.com/africa-trust-stamp-covid-19-vaccine-record-payment-system/269346/

Mystery as 57 Fishermen Test Positive for Coronavirus despite Spending 35 days at Sea and Testing negative Defore They Left
https://www.dailymail.co.uk/news/article-8520485/Mystery-57-Argentine-fishermen-test-positive-coronavirus-35-days-sea.html

Conclusive Proof — Masks Do Not Inhibit Viral Spread
https://articles.mercola.com/sites/articles/archive/2020/07/19/are-face-masks-effective.aspx?cid_source=dnl&cid_medium=email&cid_content=art1ReadMore&cid=20200719Z1

UN Unleashes Army of Trolls to Shut Down Opposition
https://articles.mercola.com/sites/articles/archive/2020/07/21/un-unleashes-army-of-trolls-to-shut-down-opposition.aspx?cid_source=dnl&cid_medium=email&cid_content=art2ReadMore&cid=20200721Z1

COVID-19 Vaccines: Hope or Hype?
http://coconutresearchcenter.org/hwnl_18-1.htm

References

Chapter 1: The Outbreak
1. https://www.cdc.gov/flu/about/burden-averted/2017-2018. htm.
2. https://articles.mercola.com/sites/articles/ archive/2020/06/17/nursing-home-deaths-from-covid-19. aspx?cid_source=dnl&cid_medium=email&cid_content=a rt3ReadMore&cid=20200617Z1&et_cid=DM567253&et_ rid=896079971.
3. https://thetruthaboutcancer.com/cdc-inflates-coronavirus-deaths/.
4. https://www.cdc.gov/nchs/nvss/vsrr/covid_weekly/index. htm.

Chapter 3: Origin of COVID-19
1. https://www.who.int/emergencies/diseases/novel-coronavirus-2019/question-and-answers-hub/q-a-detail/q-a-coronaviruses.
2. https://www.the-scientist.com/news-opinion/ modelers-struggle-to-predict-the-future-of-the-covid-19-pandemic-67261.
3. https://www.imperial.ac.uk/media/imperial-college/ medicine/sph/ide/gida-fellowships/Imperial-College-COVID19-NPI-modelling-16-03-2020.pdf.
4. https://www.livescience.com/coronavirus-outbreak-end. html.

5. https://en.wikipedia.org/wiki/COVID-19_pandemic_cases.

Chapter 4: The Coronavirus
1. Banerjee, A, et al. Bats and coronaviruses. *Viruses* 2019;11:41.
2. Lau, SK, et al. Ecoepidemiology and complete genome comparison of different strains of severe acute respiratory syndrome-related Rhinolophus bat coronavirus in China reveal bats as a reservoir for acute, self-limiting infection that allows recombination events. J Virol 2010;84:2808-2819.
3. Zumla, A, et al. Middle East respiratory syndrome.*Lancet* 2015;386:995-1007.
4. Corman, VM, et al. Link of a ubiquitous human coronavirus to dromedary camels. PNAS 2016; 201604472 DOI: 10.1073/pnas.1604472113.
5. https://www.theguardian.com/science/2014/dec/04/-sp-100-safety-breaches-uk-labs-potentially-deadly-diseases.
6. https://www.cidrap.umn.edu/news-perspective/2016/07/federal-report-discloses-incidents-high-containment-labs.
7. https://besacenter.org/perspectives-papers/china-biological-warfare/.
8. http://archive.is/tokgj.
9. https://www.wionews.com/world/chinas-bat-woman-shi-zhengli-goes-missing-297076.
10. Sanger, DE. Pompeo ties coronavirus to China lab, despite spy agencies' Uncertainty. *New York Times* May 3, 2020.]
11. Myers, SL. China spins tale that the US army started the coronavirus epidemic. *New York Times* March 13, 2020.
12. https://www.scmp.com/news/china/society/article/3052966/chinese-laboratory-first-shared-coronavirus-genome-world-ordered.
13. https://nypost.com/2020/04/15/fauci-endorses-tinder-hookups-with-a-caveat/.
14. https://www.ncbi.nlm.nih.gov/pmc/articles/PMC545012/.

15. https://www.newsweek.com/dr-fauci-backed-controversial-wuhan-lab-millions-us-dollars-risky-coronavirus-research-1500741.

Chapter 5: Fear and Panic

1. https://www.naturalproductsglobal.com/featured/natural-health-sites-blame-google-censorship-for-plummeting-web-traffic/.
2. https://www.devex.com/news/un-enlists-10-000-digital-volunteers-to-fight-covid-19-misinformation-97615#. XwSSFB1ro20.twitter.
3. https://www.npr.org/2020/05/08/852435761/as-hospitals-lose-revenue-thousands-of-health-care-workers-face-furloughs-layoff.
4. Klompas, M, et al. Universal masking in hospital in the COVID-19 era. *N Engl J Med* 2020; 382:e63 DOI: 10.1056/NEJMp2006372.
5. https://vixra.org/abs/2006.0044.
6. https://www.timesofisrael.com/the-end-of-exponential-growth-the-decline-in-the-spread-of-coronavirus/.
7. https://www.cdc.gov/nchs/data/nvss/vsrg/vsrg03-508.pdf.
8. https://townhall.com/columnists/johnrlottjr/2020/05/16/the-us-is-dramatically-overcounting-coronavirus-deaths-n2568925.
9. https://crimeresearch.org/2020/05/cross-country-data-on-coronavirus-very-problematic-in-making-comparisons-us-hospitals-paid-more-for-labeling-cause-of-death-as-coronavirus/.
10. https://www.zerohedge.com/geopolitical/several-florida-labs-report-positivity-rates-100?utm_source=feedburner&utm_medium=feed&utm_campaign=Feed%3A+zerohedge%2Ffeed+%28zero+hedge+-+on+a+long+enough+timeline%2C+the+survival+rate+for+everyone+drops+t.

Chapter 6: Are Drugs and Vaccines the Answer?

1. https://www.newswise.com/coronavirus/vitamin-d-determines-severity-in-covid-19-so-

government-advice-needs-to-change/?article_
id=731477&sc=dwhr&xy=10023815 .

2. https://www.ncbi.nlm.nih.gov/pmc/articles/
PMC7231123/.

3. Cannell, JJ, Vieth R, Umhau JC, et al. Epidemic influenza and vitamin D. *Epidemiol Infect* 2006;134:1129–1140.

4. D'Avolio, A, et al. 25-hydroxyvitamin D concentrations are lower in patients with positive PCR for SARS-CoV-2. *Nutrients* 2020;12:1359.

5. Ilie, PC, et al. The role of vitamin D in the prevention of coronavirus disease 2019 infection and mortality. *Aging Clin Exp Res* 2020, doi.org/10.1007/s40520-020-01570-8.

6. https://www.researchsquare.com/article/rs-21211/v1.

7. http://orthomolecular.activehosted.com/index.php?action
=social&chash=b73ce398c39f506af761d2277d853a92.164
&s=b5a4d78a62acf8d7d34cf4c3d0c1905f.

8. https://www.ncbi.nlm.nih.gov/pmc/articles/
PMC7137406/.

9. te Velthuis, AJW, et al. Zn2+ inhibits coronavirus and arterivirus RNA polymerase activity in vitro and zinc ionophores block the replication of these viruses in cell culture. *PLoS Pathogens* 2010; https://doi.org/10.1371/
journal.ppat.1001176.

10. https://www.youtube.com/watch?time_
continue=19&v=-oh9Ztgjm4A&feature=emb_title.

11. https://www.fox2detroit.com/news/fbi-raids-shelby-
townships-allure-medical-spa-thursday-morning.

12. https://www.wsj.com/articles/world-health-coronavirus-
disinformation-11586122093.

13. https://www.businessinsider.com/who-no-need-for-
healthy-people-to-wear-face-masks-2020-4.

14. https://www.ncbi.nlm.nih.gov/pmc/articles/
PMC1232869/.

15. https://www.ncbi.nlm.nih.gov/pmc/articles/
PMC4182877/#:~:text=Zinc%20binding%20
compounds%2C%20especially%20zinc,been%20
recently%20realized%20%5B18%5D.

16. https://www.ncbi.nlm.nih.gov/pmc/articles/
PMC3722327/

17. https://www.ncbi.nlm.nih.gov/pmc/articles/PMC3791327/.

18. https://www.cnn.com/2020/06/04/health/retraction-coronavirus-studies-lancet-nejm/index.html.

19. https://www.henryford.com/news/2020/07/hydro-treatment-study.

20. Million, M, et al. early treatment of COVID-19 patients with hydroxychloroquine and azithromycin: A retrospective analysis of 1061 cases in Marseille, France. *Travel Medicine and Infectious Disease* 2020; https://doi.org/10.1016/j.tmaid.2020.101738.

21. https://www.preprints.org/manuscript/202007.0025/v1.

22. https://thevaccinereaction.org/2020/05/volunteer-describes-his-serious-reaction-in-modernas-mrna-covid-19-vaccine-trial/.

23. https://thevaccinereaction.org/2020/07/81-percent-of-clinical-trial-volunteers-suffer-reactions-to-cansino-biologics-covid-19-vaccine-that-uses-hek293-human-fetal-cell-lines/.

24. https://articles.mercola.com/sites/articles/archive/2020/05/31/is-there-a-vaccine-for-coronavirus.aspx.

25. https://thevaccinereaction.org/2020/06/covid-19-vaccine-will-likely-be-given-multiple-times-perhaps-annually/.

26. Wang, Y, et al. Remdesivir in adults with severe COVID-19: a randomised, double-blind, placebo-controlled, multicentre trial. Lancet 2020;395:1569-1578.

27. Grein, J, et al. Compassionate use of remdesivir for patients with severe COVID-19. N Engl J Med 2020; 382:2327-2336.

28. Beigel, JH, et al. Remdesivir for the treatment of COVID-19—preliminary report. *N Engl J Med* 2020; DOI: 10.1056/NEJMoa2007764.

29. https://www.bmj.com/content/369/bmj.m2456.

30. https://theprint.in/health/govt-reviewing-remdesivir-use-for-covid-after-hospitals-report-liver-damage-in-patients/454169/?amp&__twitter_impression=true.

31. Dubert, M, et al. Case reports study of the first five patients COVID-19 treated with remdesivir in France. *International Journal of Infectious Diseases* 2020; https://doi.org/10.1016/j.ijid.2020.06.093.

Chapter 7: Who is Behind the Pandemic?

1. https://www.lifesitenews.com/news/bill-gates-life-wont-go-back-to-normal-until-population-widely-vaccinated.
2. http://blogs.reuters.com/mediafile/2008/12/01/newshour-gets-35-million-from-gates-foundation/.
3. https://www.gavi.org/our-alliance/market-shaping.
4. https://www.gatesfoundation.org/media-center/press-releases/2012/01/private-and-public-partners-unite-to-combat-10-neglected-tropical-diseases-by-2020.
5. https://www.gatesfoundation.org/How-We-Work/Quick-Links/Grants-Database/Grants/2017/11/OPP1180343.
6. https://www.gatesfoundation.org/Media-Center/Press-Releases/2020/04/Gates-Foundation-Expands-Commitment-to-COVID-19-Response-Calls-for-International-Collaboration.
7. https://www.who.int/about/finances-accountability/reports/A72_INF5-en.pdf.
8. https://archive.is/vgOWw.
9. https://www.gardenstatefamilies.org/post/covid-19-bill-gates-and-nj-pharma-is-the-gates-foundation-self-dealing.
10. https://wellbeingtrust.org/areas-of-focus/policy-and-advocacy/reports/projected-deaths-of-despair-during-covid-19/.
11. https://ips-dc.org/billionaire-bonanza-2020/.
12. https://inequality.org/billionaire-bonanza-2020-updates/
13. https://www.jnj.com/johnson-johnson-announces-a-lead-vaccine-candidate-for-covid-19-landmark-new-partnership-with-u-s-department-of-health-human-services-and-commitment-to-supply-one-billion-vaccines-worldwide-for-emergency-pandemic-use.
14. https://www.statnews.com/2020/05/19/vaccine-experts-say-moderna-didnt-produce-data-critical-to-assessing-covid-19-vaccine/.

15. https://www.forbes.com/sites/
giacomotognini/2020/05/04/these-healthcare-
billionaires-have-gotten-richer-off-the-coronavirus-
pandemic/#18e6ea8461ba.
16. https://www.fool.com/investing/2020/06/28/is-it-too-
late-to-buy-moderna-stock.aspx.
17. https://www.thestreet.com/investing/gileads-remdesivir-
bank-of-america-cautious.
18. https://www.drugs.com/news/covid-19-remdesivir-
could-cost-up-3-120-per-patient-maker-says-91171.
html?utm_source=ddc&utm_medium=email&utm_
campaign=Daily+Mednews+-+June+30%2C+2020&utm_
content=COVID-19+Drug+Remdesivir+Could+Cost+Up+t
o+%243%2C120+Per+Patient%2C+Maker+Says.
19. https://www.citizen.org/article/the-real-story-of-
remdesivir/.
20. https://www.nature.com/articles/nbt.3488.
21. https://www.statnews.com/2016/09/13/moderna-
therapeutics-biotech-mrna/.
22. https://en.wikipedia.org/wiki/Theranos.

Chapter 8: How Dangerous is COVID-19?

1. Li, R, et al. Substantial undocumented infection facilitates
the rapid dissemination of novel coronavirus (SARS-CoV2).
Science 2020; eabb3221.
2. https://www.cdc.gov/flu/about/burden/2018-2019.html#:~
:text=Conclusion,2012%E2%80%932013%20influenza%20
season1..
3. https://www.cdc.gov/flu/about/burden/preliminary-in-
season-estimates.htm.
4. https://www.spiked-online.com/2020/06/26/the-
lockdown-is-causing-so-many-deaths/.
5. https://www.cdc.gov/mmwr/volumes/69/wr/mm6912e2.
htm?s_cid=mm6912e2_w.
6. https://usa.greekreporter.com/2020/06/27/up-to-300-
million-people-may-be-infected-by-covid-19-stanford-guru-
john-ioannidis-says/.
7. https://www.spiked-online.com/2020/06/26/the-
lockdown-is-causing-so-many-deaths/amp/?__twitter_
impression=true.

8. https://mailchi.mp/tomwoods/upmc?e=6d5eb520c3.

9. https://off-guardian.org/2020/06/12/study-80-of-people-naturally-resistant-to-coronavirus/.

10. https://www.researchsquare.com/article/rs-35331/v1.

11. https://www.sciencemag.org/news/2020/05/t-cells-found-covid-19-patients-bode-well-long-term-immunity.

12. https://www.biorxiv.org/content/10.1101/2020.05.26.115832v1.full.pdf.

13. https://www.cell.com/cell/fulltext/S0092-8674(20)30610-3#.XtUNRAVlzFA.twitter.

14. https://www.cdc.gov/coronavirus/2019-ncov/testing/serology-overview.html.

Chapter 9: A Misinformation Campaign

1. Li, R, et al. Substantial undocumented infection facilitates the rapid dissemination of novel coronavirus (SARS-CoV-2). *Science* 2020; eabb3221.

2. https://www.cnbc.com/2020/06/08/asymptomatic-coronavirus-patients-arent-spreading-new-infections-who-says.html.

3. https://mailchi.mp/tomwoods/upmc?e=6d5eb520c3.

4. https://www.dailymail.co.uk/news/article-8425671/Two-metre-rule-NO-basis-science-leading-scientists-say-amid-calls-drop-measure.html.

5. https://www.cnbc.com/2020/05/06/ny-gov-cuomo-says-its-shocking-most-new-coronavirus-hospitalizations-are-people-staying-home.html.

6. Hobday, RA and Cason, JW. The open-air treatment of pandemic influenza. *Am J Public Health* 2009;99(Suppl 2);S236-S242.

7. Cook, GC. Early use of "open-air" treatment for "pulmonary phthisis" at the Dreadnought Hospital, Greenwich, 1900–1905. *Postgrad Med J* 1999;75:326–327.

8. Anon. Influenza at the Camp Brooks Open Air Hospital. *JAMA* 1918;71:1746–1747.

9. Hill, LE. The defence of the respiratory membrane against influenza, etc. *Br Med J* 1919;1:238–240.

10. Anon. Weapons against influenza. *Am J Public Health* 1918;8:787–788.

11. Brooks, WA. The open air treatment of influenza. *Am J Public Health* 1918;8:746–750.

12. Sagripanti JL, Lytle CD. Inactivation of influenza virus by solar radiation. *Photochem Photobiol* 2007;83:1278–1282.

13. Sagripanti, JL and Lytle, CD. Estimated inactivation of coronaviruses by solar radiation with special reference to COVID-19. *Photochem Photobiol* 2020 Jun 5;10.1111/php.13293. doi: 10.1111/php.13293.

14. https://www.eatthis.com/coronavirus-sun-protection/.

15. https://www.worldometers.info/coronavirus/country/us/.

16. https://www.aier.org/article/an-egregious-statistical-horror-story-suffused-with-incense-and-lugubrious-accents/?fbclid=IwAR1NJlw4fINXTw__Ki8lrXajCVTYvl4FIlnURVAzHo-EldUCzYLH9egKs5Q.

Index

Qiu, Xiangguo, 30
Quarantine, 41, 81
Quercetin, 48

Raccoon dog, 27
Rancourt, Dennis, 43
Raoult, Didier, 54
Remdesivir, 61-64, 73-75
Rhinovirus, 24, 86
Risch, Harvey, 55-56
RNA viruses, 75

Sanatorium, 93
SARS-CoV (SARS), 17,
  18-19, 21, 25-26
SARS-Cov-2, 17, 21-23,
  25, 29-36, 48, 60, 86
Schaffner, William, 23, 59
Shapiro, Steven, 85
Social distancing, 16, 40-
  44, 92-93, 98, 104

Social media, 50
Common cold, 24, 27,
  86-87
Spanish flu, 16, 40, 93
Sunshine, 93-97, 104

T cells, 86-87
Testing kits, 72
Theranos, 76
Tuberculosis, 93-94, 102

Ultraviolet light, 48
United Nations (UN), 40
USS Theodore Roosevelt,
  96-97

Vaccines, 57-61, 98-99,
  102, 103
Van Kerkhove, Maria,
  89, 91
Vitamin D, 25, 47-49, 95
Vò, 81

Wenliang, Li, 19-20
Wet market, 27-28
Wittkowski, Knut, 50
Wojcicki, Susan, 51
World Health Organiza-
  tion (WHO), 20-21, 40,
  51, 67, 101
Wuhan, 18, 29, 81
Wuhan Inistitute of
  Virology (WIV), 29, 32,
  35-36

YouTube, 39, 50, 51

Zelenko, Vlddimir, 54-55
Zhiming, Yuan, 32
Zhengli, Shi, 32, 35
Zinc, 49, 52, 53, 54
Zuckerberg, Mark, 71

www.ingramcontent.com/pod-product-compliance
Lightning Source LLC
Chambersburg PA
CBHW050530280326
41933CB00011B/1526